Griffiths III – A Case Study Book for Practitioners

Griffiths III – A Case Study Book for Practitioners

Louise Stroud
Elizabeth Green
(Editors)

hogrefe

Library of Congress of Congress Cataloging in Publication information for the print version of this book is available via the Library of Congress Marc Database under the Library of Congress Control Number 2022938521

Library and Archives Canada Cataloguing in Publication

Title: Griffiths III : a case study book for practitioners / Louise Stroud, Elizabeth Green (editors).
Other titles: Griffiths 3 | Griffiths three
Names: Stroud, Louise (Louise A.), editor. | Green, Elizabeth (Elizabeth M.), editor.
Description: Includes bibliographical references.
Identifiers: Canadiana (print) 20220238006 | Canadiana (ebook) 20220240809 | ISBN 9780889375918 (softcover) | ISBN 9781616765910 (PDF) | ISBN 9781613345917 (EPUB)
Subjects: LCSH: Child development—Testing. | LCSH: Child development—Testing—Case studies.
Classification: LCC RJ51.D48 G75 2022 | DDC 618.92/0075—dc23

www.hogrefe.com

Original illustrations on the section title pages by Sarah Stroud.

PUBLISHING OFFICES

USA:	Hogrefe Publishing Corporation, 44 Merrimac Street, Suite 207, Newburyport, MA 01950 Phone (978) 255 3700; E-mail customersupport@hogrefe.com
EUROPE:	Hogrefe Publishing GmbH, Merkelstr. 3, 37085 Göttingen, Germany Phone +49 551 99950 0, Fax +49 551 99950 111; E-mail publishing@hogrefe.com

SALES & DISTRIBUTION

USA:	Hogrefe Publishing, Customer Services Department, 30 Amberwood Parkway, Ashland, OH 44805 Phone (800) 228 3749, Fax (419) 281 6883; E-mail customersupport@hogrefe.com
UK:	Hogrefe Publishing, c/o Marston Book Services Ltd., 160 Eastern Ave., Milton Park, Abingdon, OX14 4SB Phone +44 1235 465577, Fax +44 1235 465556; E-mail direct.orders@marston.co.uk
EUROPE:	Hogrefe Publishing, Merkelstr. 3, 37085 Göttingen, Germany Phone +49 551 99950 0, Fax +49 551 99950 111; E-mail publishing@hogrefe.com

OTHER OFFICES

CANADA:	Hogrefe Publishing Corporation, 82 Laird Drive, East York, Ontario M4G 3V1
SWITZERLAND:	Hogrefe Publishing, Länggass-Strasse 76, 3012 Bern

Printed and bound in the Czech Republic

ISBN 978-0-88937-591-8 (print) · ISBN 978-1-61676-591-0 (PDF) · ISBN 978-1-61334-591-7 (EPUB)
http://doi.org/10.1027/00591-000

In Memory of Our Friend and Colleague

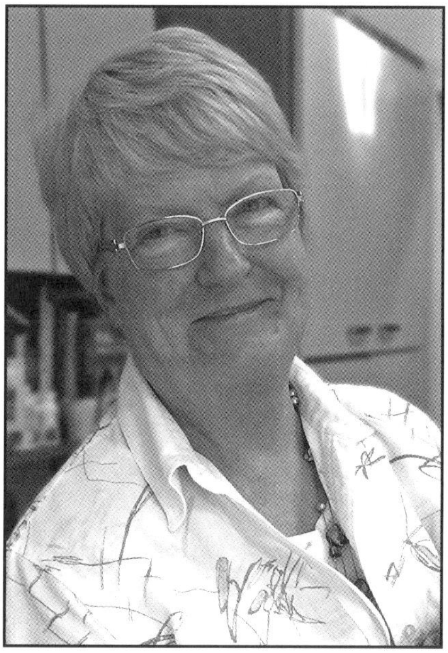

Rosemary O’Connell
(July 8, 1946–July 16, 2021)

Contents

About the Editors

Louise Stroud, PhD, is a registered clinical psychologist and full professor employed in the Department of Psychology of the Faculty of Health Sciences at the Nelson Mandela University in Port Elizabeth, South Africa. She is also the lead researcher for the Association for Research in Infant and Child Development (ARICD, https://www.aricd.ac.uk/) based in Manchester, UK. Her specific research interests include the study of the psychology of people and their lives, the development of children, neuropsychology, and ecopsychology.

Elizabeth Green, MD, is a retired developmental pediatrician, former consultant in pediatric rehabilitation at Chailey Heritage Clinical Services, former medical director of South Downs Health NHS Trust in Brighton, and past president of ARICD. She currently holds the research chair and is a trustee of ARICD. She is also a trustee of the Chailey Heritage Foundation and research associate at the Psychology Department at the Nelson Mandela University in South Africa.

Foreword

While we try to teach our children all about life,
our children teach us what life is all about.

– Angela Schwindt

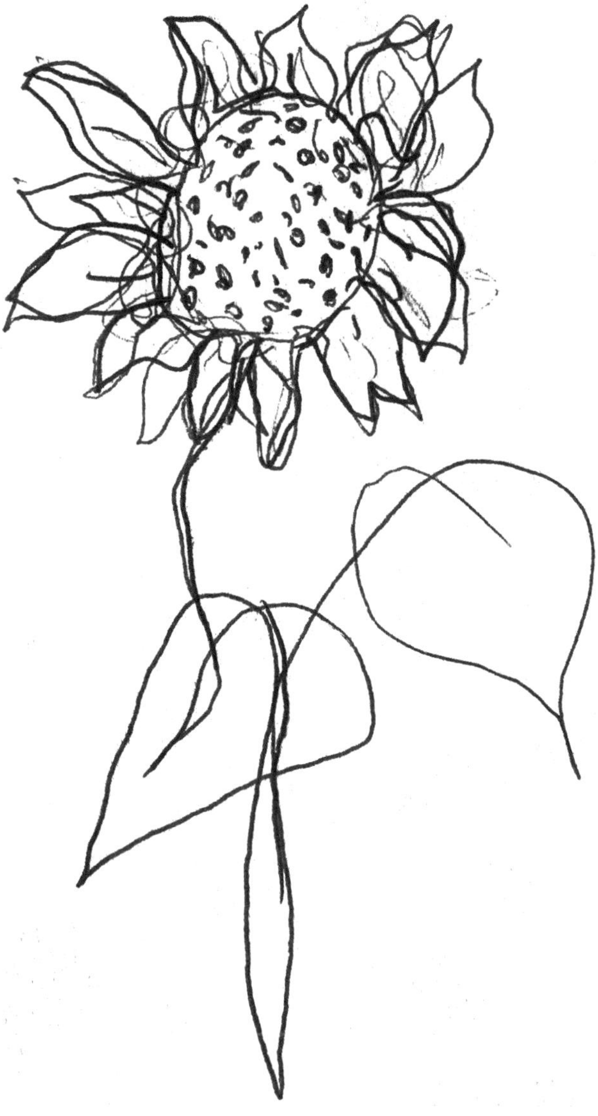

Illustrations by Sarah Stroud

The publication of *Griffiths III – A Case Study Book for Practitioners* in 2022 as the world begins to emerge from the ravages of the Covid-19 pandemic could not be timelier. Many lessons have and will be learnt from the pandemic, but the precious lesson that children need both play and school to flourish must never be forgotten. While children were mercifully far less impacted by the virus itself, we have learnt hard lessons about how children can be affected when school is delivered online, when play and sport are no longer possible, when meeting up with friends is prohibited, and when routine and life as it is known stop.

Our children have shown remarkable resilience and courage in the last two years, but we know that not all have come through unscathed. Children from the most socially disadvantaged communities and children with health and developmental problems have paid a heavy price, and so it is these groups that need specific focus, care, and attention as we recover from the pandemic.

The problems that face us can feel daunting. However, many of the solutions we need come very simply from listening to the children and families we serve. Children and young people have been articulate and engaged – both in describing the problems as they see them, but then also crucially in showing us where the solutions lie. The children and young people who work with the Royal College of Paediatrics and Child Health, RCPCH&Us, have been very clear about what they believe mental health services should look like, how virtual consultations should be set up, and crucially how they want to be central to service planning and development. Fundamentally, our children are telling us they have a voice, and they want to be listened to and valued.

Louise Stroud and Elizabeth Green have done a masterful job of placing the child at the center of this book, and the voice of children and their families ring through the pages. This is not a simple training manual on how to undertake the Griffiths III, a standardized test. This book is so much more: It makes the clear case for treating each child and each family as a unique entity. It consistently emphasizes why it is crucial to adapt and modify how the test is undertaken and interpreted to the context of the child in the moment. Stroud and Green achieve what every pediatrician hopes to achieve in each clinical encounter – the child is considered in the context of their health, family, education, social situation, and so much more. Crucially, they make the case for acknowledging and celebrating diversity – diversity of culture, parenting, socio-economic background, and more.

I commend this book to all who work in the field of child development and more widely with children who are not following a typical developmental pathway. Hearing the voice of the child in all we do and underpinning our work with compassion and kindness should be fundamental. This book will help you achieve that.

Camilla Kingdon, MA MBChB FRCPCH
Consultant Neonatologist, Guy's and St Thomas' NHS Foundation Trust
President of Royal College of Paediatrics and Child Health
London, UK

Preface

Louise Stroud and Elizabeth Green

Oh, the Places You'll Go! is the last children's book Dr. Seuss authored (Geisel, 1990), and it is his guide to the journey of life. It is a brief story that reminds us that we can be the things we want to be, with a little bit of work and will power. Without ignoring the basic fact of life that everything does not always go ideally, the book encourages us to get out there and make things happen. According to Dr. Seuss, waiting for something to happen is the worst choice that anyone can make; for nothing can be gained, if nothing is risked. Similarly, Pierre van der Merwe in his book *The Adventures of Auggy (Book Two): The Magic Lily Pad* tells the story of Auggy, a very popular little froggy, who lived in a pond. Legend had it that if Auggy, or anyone for that matter, saw the magic lily-pad on the pond and made a wish, their wish would come true. The magic lily-pad got its name from the reflection of the sun and moon on the pond which became like golden and silver lily-pads, as the sun and moon moved across the pond. The message behind the story of Auggy and the magic lily-pad is that there is still magic even when everything is not what one would want or think it to be (Babb & van der Merwe, 1997). These two children's stories provide a lovely start to this Griffiths III Case Study Book for Practitioners. Their messages of courage, will power, risk, and believing in magic are most appropriate not only for the practitioner with an interest in children and their development, but also for the children they serve.

This Case Book is a professional reference book. Although aimed particularly at Griffiths III practitioners, it will also be of interest to a wide range of developmental practitioners. The approach taken in this book is to use individual case studies to demonstrate how Griffiths III can be used in a comprehensive assessment of a child's development, of their strengths and their needs. It aims to offer practitioners practical examples of the application of aspects of Griffiths III beyond simple first-level training, to administer test items correctly. It also meets the need to clarify how the test may be used with a nontypical population.

It must be said that compiling this Case Book did not involve a description or story that fell easily and smoothly into sequence. It was a process that was garnered from many sources and from many people. Some of the Case Book comes in the form of fragments from professional men and women who have looked on developing children, with a unique and unrelenting eye. It comes from men and women who carry the germ of knowledge, implanted somewhere deeply in their beings, a place where a curious, natural rhythm exists and a kind of magic. It describes the interplay between universal and unique contexts in shaping child developmental assessment, specifically using Griffiths III. Ruth Griffiths described this as the sixth sense (Griffiths, 1968).

In this Case Book for Practitioners, the Griffiths Scales of Child Development, 3rd edition, or Griffiths III as it is known, will be described. Griffiths III is a test which is instrumental in determining whether a child is developing age appropriately, or whether a general or specific developmental difficulty is indicated. Griffiths III is used in the assessment of all children but particularly in the assessment of children with disabilities and the creation of appropriate intervention plans. Practitioners need to understand the test to formulate it successfully with a child with disability. To this end they have asked for a practical book with examples to deepen their understanding of the test and clarify how the test may be used with a nontypical population.

The assessment of development involves a comprehensive investigation of a child's abilities, including motor, social, and cognitive abilities, by direct observation, testing, and reports from caregivers. The rapidly shifting nature of children's development poses problems for the assessment of young children. Of the various methods for assessing child development, Griffiths III is among those that have been accorded world-wide recognition, especially by pediatricians and psychologists. It is not simply a screening test, for it enables a thorough, holistic diagnosis through analysis of the developmental profile. Through periodic reexaminations of children, we can bring to light developmental trends and establish developmental baselines.

In the past, the *working child* toiled in the fields, and later, in the factories of the Industrial Revolution. The 20th century saw the rise of the *free-range child,* and more recently we have experienced the emergence of the age of the *managed child* with the *helicopter parent* hovering overhead trying to control things. Today, more specifically, we face the challenge of finding a new recipe for assessment of children growing up in the information age. However, regardless of the period of time in which they find themselves, children thrive when they have time and space to breathe, to chill and get bored sometimes, to relax, to take risks and make mistakes, to dream and have fun on their own terms, even to fail. Their appetite for change leads them to be curious about the world about them. They love to play. They need to play. It connects them to the real world – their real world.

Nell and Drew (2013) state that children learn to make their own decisions when they play and experience freedom in making those choices. They begin to see connections between choice and the consequences or results of that choice, this inspires creative thinking and delight. Because children eventually find it more important to be part of play with their friends than to satisfy their own wants and needs at that moment, children learn self-control. And self-control has been shown to lead to success in later years, especially in today's information age, where distractions are part of daily life. Play provides children with opportunities to develop flexibility in their thinking and decision making, which is a vital life skill.

Play is a science and an essential ingredient in optimal child development. It has been described as a lighting up of the brain. The Griffiths Scales are not play-based scales but have been structured since Ruth Griffiths' first publication to include the types of play children enjoy at different stages of their development. Because children are intrinsically motivated to enjoy play, observing a child performing a structured activity in a play context offers much more information about the child's strengths and any barriers to development than a simple pass/fail.

All children should have equal access to play, which is fundamental to childhood, and yet it has been found that disabled children have significantly fewer opportunities to access, and more barriers to, play settings and activities than their nondisabled peers. According to Sense's website resource *Making Play Inclusive: A Toolkit for Play Settings* (https://www.sense.org.uk/get-support/support-for-children/play-toolkits/), the key principles for inclusive play include the following:

- Equality does not mean treating everyone the same; it is about making the adjustments that enable all children to take part.

- Every child is unique. It is important to take the time to get to know each child, prepare for and understand their needs, and know where to go for further advice.
- Give children time to respond, explore, and play.
- A can-do attitude is really important – always focus on what the child can do and understand what achievement means for each child.
- Manage risk effectively; don't let it get in the way of play.
- Listen, discuss, plan, and consult with parents.
- Where possible, treatments and therapeutic interventions should be delivered through play.

As practitioners with an interest in child development, it is necessary for us to establish children's developmental baselines as well as their individual barriers to development. For example, in the past this need led the developmental psychologist Plooij to speak of *regression periods*, the child neuropsychologist Vygotsky to highlight the importance of *zones of proximal development*, the cognitive psychologist Piaget to suggest that cognitive development progresses as change happens in the child's knowledge systems, and the child psychologist Ruth Griffiths to create the Griffiths Scales of Child Development.

Dr. Ruth Florence Griffiths was born on September 2, 1895. She experienced an isolated and troubled childhood (which she seemed to remember forever after). Dr. Brian Burne records that it was perhaps these early experiences that laid the roots for her later meticulous observation of young children, her love for them, and her pleasure in observing their personalities unfold and blossom. J. C. Flugel also referred to Griffith's observation of the free behavior of children, her rigorous control of experimental conditions, and her ingenuity, tact, and perseverance, as being full of promise for the future. How right he was, as Griffiths went on to design and create the Griffiths Scales which were published in 1954.

When the Griffiths Scales were first introduced, the psychometric conceptions of intelligence were emerging and were to influence psychometric measurement for the next three generations. These narrow conceptions included verbal, visual-spatial, and mathematical abilities. The Griffiths Scales brought with them an innovative system for developmental assessment, as Griffiths was keenly aware of the importance of interactions between the various avenues of learning. She advocated a broad-based approach to understanding development (i.e., the processes and rates at which growth and maturation of a child's attributes and abilities take place) and the concept of the observation of children in play. She was aware of the importance of social and emotional developmental factors and the interplay between these and development.

This Case Book puts the perspective of the child at the center and considers their voices. It considers their identities and developmental stages. It embraces their agency through promoting advocacy. It does not distrust or discount other voices, such as those of adult experts, but rather seeks to fulfill the child's need to be heard within the considerations of barriers that may challenge the fulfillment of this right. This is a deliberate and reflexive account of the child's story within a context of diversity. It is an acknowledgement of the agency of children and the insertion of their voices into their stories, while being guided by their accounts of their lives, and the accounts of their lives by others. In essence, this is an insider–outsider approach, which makes for a child-centric Case Book for Practitioners using Griffiths III. It aims to assist practitioners to better track and monitor development, plan and measure the impact of intervention, and inform decisions about management and placement of the child. It hopes to aid in the creation of a community of practice among

Griffiths III users worldwide. A place where the voices of the children we assess are listened to and heard. The Chinese symbol for "listen" captures this most aptly, as it is made up of four parts – namely, the ears, the eyes, the heart, and undivided attention. This is reflected visually below:

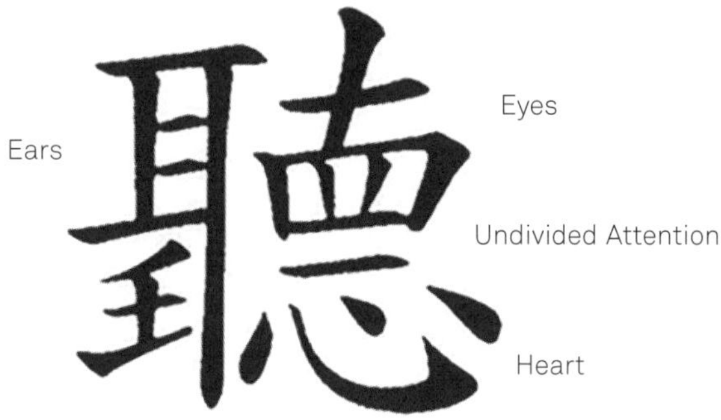

References

Babb, N., & van der Merwe, P. (1997). *The adventures of Auggy. Book Two: The magic Lily-Pad*. Young Edwards.

Geisel, T. S. (Dr. Seuss). (1990). *Oh the places you'll go!* HarperCollins.

Griffiths, R. (1968). The psycho-diagnostic approach to problems of the very young. In E. Miller (Ed.), *Foundations of child psychiatry*. Pergomon Press.

Nell, M. L., & Drew, W. F. (2013). *From play to practice: Connecting teachers' play to childrens' learning*. The National Association for the Education of Young Children.

Section I

Introduction

All you need to know about children for children – you learn best from them!

– Loris Malaguzzi

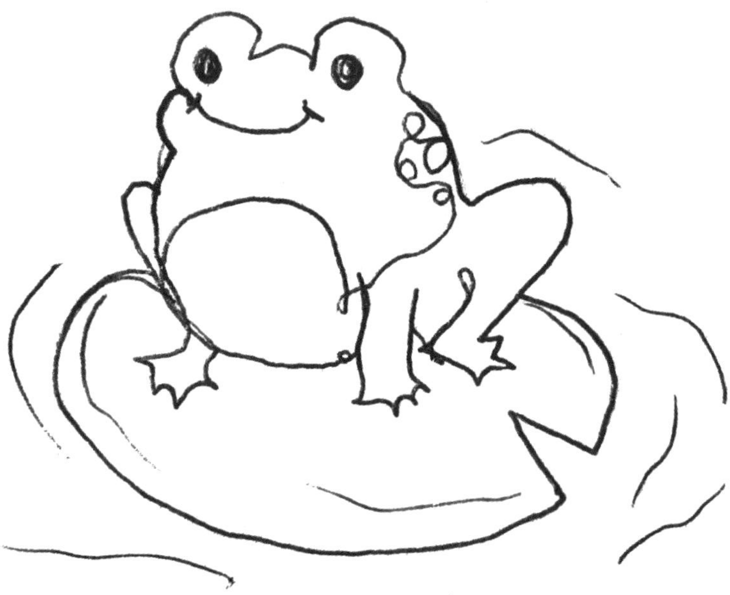

Chapter 1

An Introduction to the Griffiths III Case Study Book

Louise Stroud and Elizabeth Green

Why a Griffiths III Case Study Book?

Griffiths III is a standardized test, but every child is unique. Any adaptations must be personal to each child. It is necessary to look at patterns of behavior, skills, and needs, and how the *avenues of learning* (Griffiths, 1954) fulfill current biopsychosocial-environmental perspectives within the disability field.

Purpose of the Case Study Book

The aim of this book is to offer practitioners practical examples of the application of aspects of Griffiths III beyond simple first-level training, to administer test items correctly. It will also meet the need for publishers to clarify how the test may be used with a nontypical population. Furthermore, amplifying children's voices, advocating for their protection and agency, and representing them in a way that is fair and eliminates injustices are all parts of the important groundwork necessary for fine-tuning and ensuring the rights of children in every respect.

Multiprofessional and Multiprocess Context of the Case Study Book

Most children who are assessed with Griffiths III have a number of people on their "team." This includes the child's family and often a multiprofessional team from education and health services. Their perspectives on the child's developmental strengths and needs are a vital part of the assessment. Their input into what they need from the assessment is also important both to consider the implications of the assessment for the child, family, and their wider environment, and to design a useful intervention plan.

Four Conceptual Frameworks

This book has four underlying conceptual frameworks which are used as a foundation throughout the book. A summary of those is shown in Figure 1.1 (a summary of the concepts and measurements used in the case studies, noted by chapter, is to be found in Tables A1 and A2 in the Appendix).

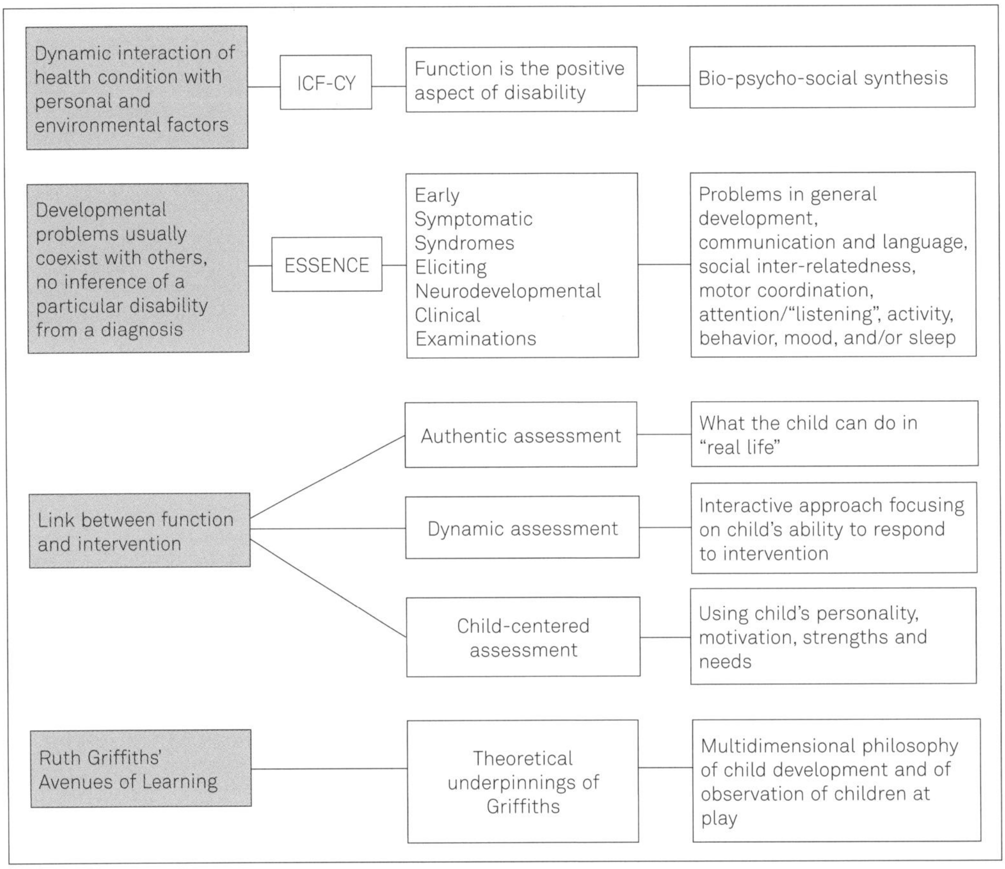

Figure 1.1. Four conceptual frameworks. ESSENCE = Early Symptomatic Syndromes Eliciting Neurodevelopmental Clinical Examinations; ICY-CF = *International Classification of Functioning, Disability and Health of Children and Youth*

Framework One: The ICY-CF

The *International Classification of Functioning, Disability and Health of Children and Youth* (ICF-CY; WHO, 2007) follows an approach in which data collected on the child are interpreted more widely, and it includes all those people who know the child in their different contexts. In this manner, a more complete profile of the lived experience of having a disability and its impact on daily life and activities is obtained. It is a version of the

International Classification of Functioning, Disability and Health (ICF; WHO, 2001) that is designed to be appropriate for children, especially those with disabilities. The paradigm shift from a medical to a broader biopsychosocial model of disability, including a modeling of the child-environment interaction as dimensions of disability, led to the consideration of an approach consistent within a framework of children's rights. This biopsychosocial model of disability was developed in the practices for children and the development of measures to capture profiles of individual differences of children. The extent to which factors in the person's environment have a facilitating or hindering effect is considered, and the ICF-CY describes both the nature and severity of the limitations of a child's functioning and also identifies the environmental factors influencing such functioning.

Framework Two: ESSENCE

In this framework, the Early Symptomatic Syndromes Eliciting Neurodevelopmental Clinical Examinations (ESSENCE) of a child are carefully considered. The importance of having a broad view in the assessments of children with developmental deviations has been emphasized by Gillberg (2010). The concept highlights the fact that many disorders, such as attention deficit/hyperactivity disorder (also known as ADHD), oppositional defiance disorder, developmental coordination disorder, language disorder, tic disorders, and intellectual disability, may coexist in children in different combinations, and any of these may coexist with autistic spectrum disorder (ASD). Many of these disorders are also accompanied by a range of behavioral problems such as sleeping problems, feeding problems, tantrums, and sensory hypersensitivities or hyposensitivities (Carlsson et al., 2013). Levy and colleagues (2010) examined children with co-occurring non-ASD diagnoses and symptoms in a population-based cohort of 8-year-old children with ASD, who had been identified during a surveillance program. They found that 80% of these children had at least one other developmental diagnosis, and 10% had at least one other psychiatric diagnosis.

The ESSENCE approach is that all problems need to be recognized, and all interventions tailored to equip the child throughout the lifespan. Gillberg (2014) suggests that the introduction of the ESSENCE manner of thinking about a child's problems related to deviations from normal child development should not be taken as support for grouping rather than splitting, but support for the order in which these two aspects of diagnosis are approached.

The assessment of neurodevelopment, both neuropsychological and neuropsychiatric, must allow for a better understanding of the child and their "condition." In ESSENCE, overlap/comorbidity/coexistence is the rule – there is no sharp boundary, and there is always overlap. The key to creating an ESSENCE-friendly environment is finding the child's strengths and needs.

Framework Three: Dynamic, Authentic, Child-Centered Assessment

To begin with, the dynamic, authentic, child-centered assessment approach advocates a *dynamic assessment*, based on Vygotsky's sociocultural theory (Salkind, 2004). Dynamic assessment is interactive and concerns an exploration of a young person's actual (independent) level of development (and problem solving), as well as their level of proximal (or potential) development (i.e., that which is possible, given support by an adult or more experienced person). The Daffodil Project – Dynamic Assessment of Functioning Oriented at Development and Inclusive Learning is an example of the use of dynamic assessment (Lebeer et al., 2013).

Authentic assessment (Bagnato, 2007, 2009) aims to understand a child's functioning in a dynamic and interactive way; how to improve their functioning, learning, and participation; and what might be hindering participation. Authentic assessment practices are collaborative with families, and are equitable, sensitive, and congruent with child-centered practices such as appropriate materials and methods that match the child's interests and developmental level (Harvey et al., 2011).

Finally, *child-centered assessment* puts the child at the center of the learning process and meets the needs of each individual child. This means looking at things from the child's perspective, allowing them to participate in planning activities and events within society. The United Nations Convention on the Rights of the Child (1990) states that "A mentally or physically disabled child should enjoy a full and decent life in conditions which ensure dignity, promote self-reliance and facilitate the child's active participation in the community" (p. 7). Each child's individual strengths and needs should be the basis of an intervention or educational plan which is tailored to that child rather than on a curriculum designed for the majority.

Framework Four: The Avenues of Learning

Ruth Griffiths' view of child development was reflected in her philosophy based on the basic avenues of learning and the concept of observing children in play (Griffiths, 1954). It is necessary to look at patterns of behavior, skills, and needs, and how the avenues of learning fulfill the current biopsychosocial-environmental perspectives within the disability field. The two-dimensional 1954 diagram of Ruth Griffiths has been revised and transformed into a three-dimensional working model to depict the theoretical underpinnings of Griffiths III. The premise of her original notion of the avenues of learning – the observation of children engaged in play and the importance of space, rhythm, and time – has been reflected in this new model (Stroud, Marais, et al., 2016). It has three spheres: The first, innermost sphere contains the *individual* section, about the child. The second sphere represents the *interpersonal* influences on a child's development, and the third represents the *socioenvironmental* influences on a child's development. Figure 1.2 shows the contemporary model of the avenues of learning

The Griffiths subscales are now included within the diagram. These have therefore been moved from being a model which reflects only the foundation on which the Griffiths Scales were developed, to a model incorporating the manner in which Griffiths III functions. By being able to view each of the individual subscales in three dimensions along a temporal dynamic plane, it is possible to visually represent a child's performance along each subscale arrow; the use of multiple moving arrows emphasizes the dynamic nature of a child's development; and a visual representation of the tracking of a child's developmental progression over multiple assessments and years is thus possible (Stroud, Foxcroft, et al., 2016).

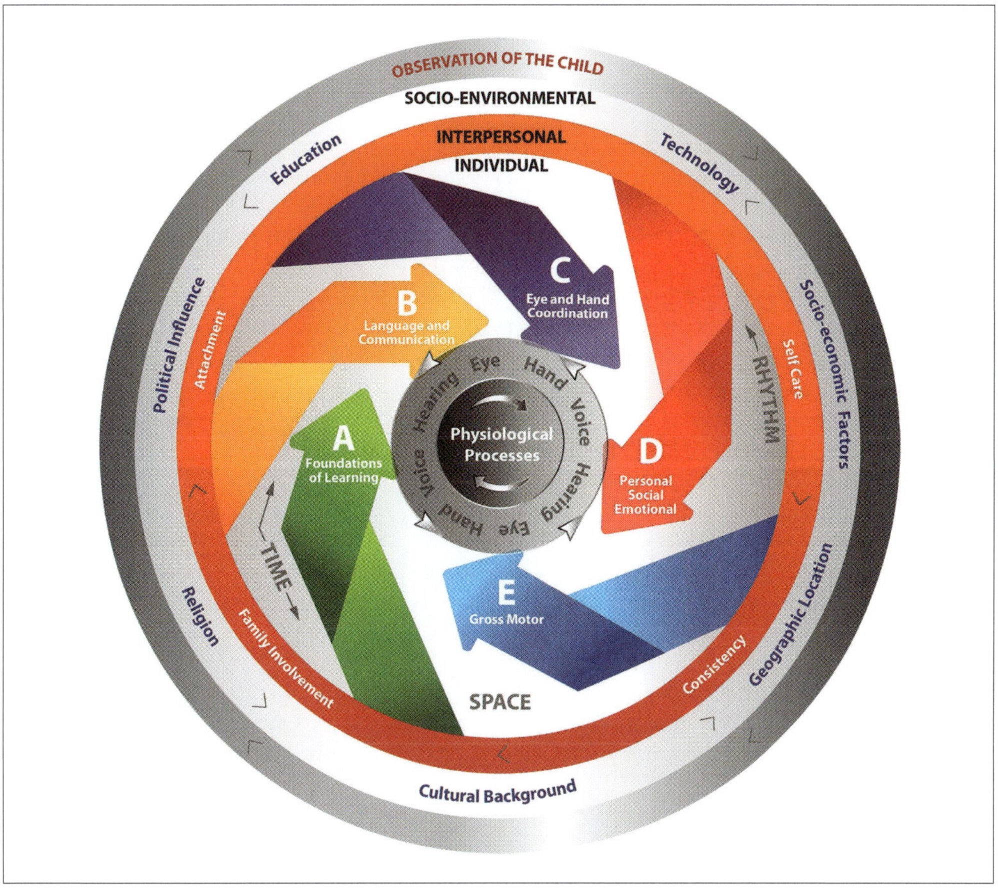

Figure 1.2. The contemporary model of the avenues of learning

Structure of the Case Study Section

The four conceptual frameworks make any classification of groupings by diagnosis no longer relevant. However, for ease of reading, some grouping is helpful. The case studies have been grouped into five colored zones.

The following section, Section II, is divided into two chapters, both of which will serve to help the practitioner understand Griffiths III as a psychological test in order to understand the child and their developmental strengths and needs and interpret their performance.

References

Bagnato, S. J. (2007). *Authentic assessment for early childhood intervention: Best practices.* Guilford Publications.

Bagnato, S. J. (2009). What are the professional standards for assessment of preschool children? In S. J. Bagnato (Ed.), *Authentic assessment for early childhood intervention: Best practices* (pp. 1–16). Guilford Press.

Carlsson, L. H., Norrelgen, F., & Fernell, E. (2013). Coexisting disorders and problems in preschool children with autistic spectrum disorders. *Scientific World Journal, 2013,* 213979, 1–6. https://doi.org/10.1155/2013/213979

Gillberg, C. (2010). The ESSENCE in child psychiatry: early symptomatic syndromes eliciting neurodevelopmental clinical examinations. *Research in Developmental Disabilities, 31*(6), 1543–1551. https://doi.org/10.1016/j.ridd.2010.06.002

Gillberg, C. (2014). *ADHD and its many associated problems.* Oxford University Press. https://doi.org/10.1093/med/9780199937905.001.0001

Griffiths, R. (1954). *The abilities of babies.* McGraw-Hill.

Harvey, H., Grisham-Brown, J., & Pretti-Frontczak, K. (2011). *Assessing young children in inclusive settings: The blended practices approach.* Paul Brookes.

Lebeer, J., Partanen, P., & Candeias, A. (2013). The need for a more dynamic and ecological assessment of children experiencing barriers to learning to move towards inclusive education: A summary of results of the Daffodil Project. *Erdélyi Pszichológiai Szemle (Transylvanian Journal of Psychology), 14,* 175–205. https://www.researchgate.net/publication/271838045

Levy, S. E., Giarelli, L. C., & Rice, C. E. (2010). Autism spectrum disorder and co-occurring developmental, psychiatric, and medical conditions among children in multiple populations of the United States. *Journal of Developmental and Behavioral Paediatrics, 31*(4), 267–275. https://doi.org/10.1097/DBP.0b013e3181d5d03b

Salkind, N. J. (2004). Lev Vygotsky's sociocultural theory of development. In *An introduction to theories of human development* (pp. 277–290). SAGE Publications. https://doi.org/10.4135/9781483328676.n10

Stroud, L., Foxcroft, C., Green, E., Bloomfield, S., Cronje, C., Hurter, K., Lane, H., Marais, R., Marx, C., McAlinden, P., O'Connell, R., Paradice, R., & Venter, D. (2016). *Griffiths III: Griffiths scales of child development. Part I: Overview, development and psychometric properties.* Hogrefe.

Stroud, L., Marais, R., & Collet, G. (2016). *Towards a contemporary Ruth Griffiths avenues of learning model* [Unpublished manuscript]. Department of Psychology, Nelson Mandela University, Port Elizabeth.

United Nations Convention on the Rights of the Child, 1990. Art. 23, Sec 1. https://www.ohchr.org/sites/default/files/crc.pdf

World Health Organization. (2001). *International classification of functioning, disability and health.*

World Health Organization. (2007). *International classification of functioning, disability and health: Children and youth version: ICF-CY.* World Health Organization. https://apps.who.int/iris/handle/10665/43737

Section II

Griffiths III – A Child Development Assessment Tool

There are no seven wonders of the world
in the eyes of a child. There are seven million.

– Walt Streightiff

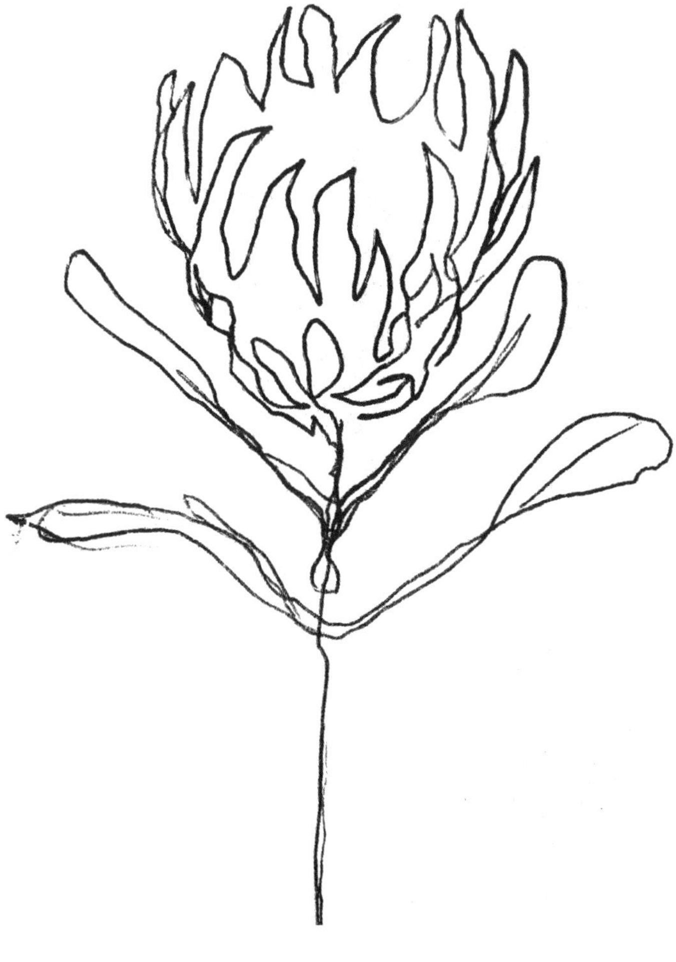

Griffiths III – A Child Development Assessment Tool

Chapter 2

Understanding the Griffiths III test properties to understand a child's performance

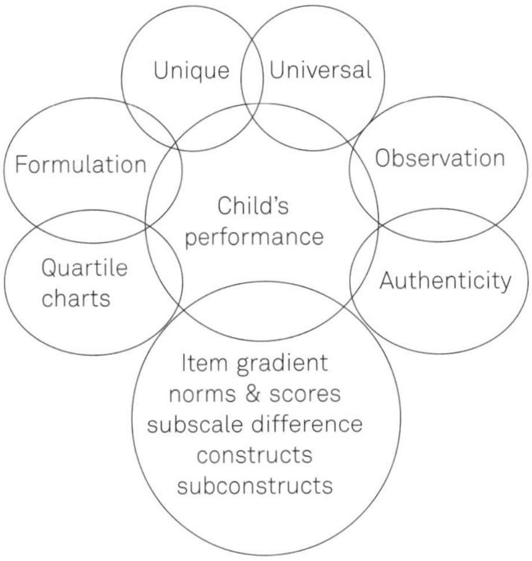

Chapter 3

Using Griffiths III to interpret, plan, and report a child's needs

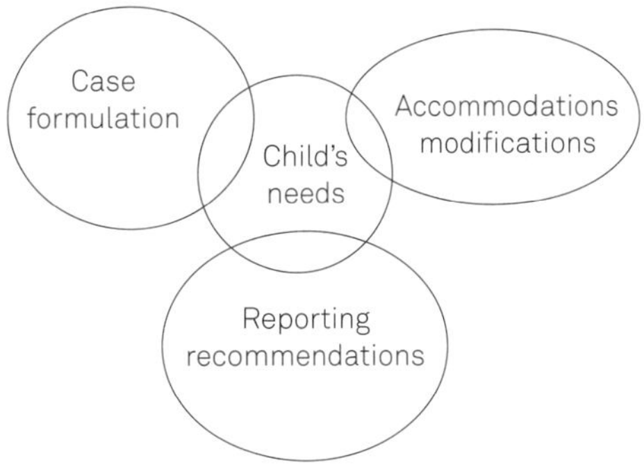

Chapter 2

Understanding the Griffiths III Test Properties to Understand a Child's Performance

Hilary Lane and Johan Cronje

This chapter outlines the variables that need to be considered when carrying out a comprehensive developmental assessment using Griffiths III. In essence, it provides an understanding of Griffiths III within the context of testing and assessment in order to better understand the child and their developmental needs

It addresses the complex nature of infants' and young children's development from the universal to the unique, and the impact of innate, environmental, and cultural influences on how assessments should be authentic and meaningful. The psychometric properties of Griffiths III are explained so clinicians can understand how to use the test to understand a child's performance and their developmental strengths and needs.

The Interplay of Universal and Unique in Every Child – The Nature of Variation and Culture

Babies' brains are designed to learn. They develop and grow by creating a complex network of connections between the billions of nerve cells they are born with. Their developing brains leave them with an uninhibited flexibility that allows them to explore, create, and learn flexibly and effectively, which is what makes each child's web of development so unique. The developing brain is influenced by innate as well as many external factors including experiences, relationships, and the environment.

Societal and cultural influences on children's development are considerable, while at the same time, children are unique with individual character strengths and abilities. Individual family interactions bring with them cultural beliefs, values, and behaviors (Maschinot, 2008). The child's ways of interacting with the people and world around them shape how they think and behave. Thus, children play an active role in their own development, which is influenced by biological factors as well as by their interactions with the environment. This has long been an underlying premise underpinning the development of the Griffiths Scales.

Recent research by both Ertem and colleagues (2018) and Villar and colleagues (2019) has confirmed that the sequence and timing of the attainment of key neurodevelopmental milestones and associated behaviors in early childhood are likely innate and universal, as long as health, nutrition, medical care, and educational needs are met. These studies advance the understanding of early childhood development by showing that many milestones in numerous domains are similarly attained across sexes and countries. Markers of neurodevelopment such as cognition, attention, language, motor, and visual capacity are fundamental human functions, and their development has been reported to reflect the rapid growth and maturation of the brain (Knickmeyer et al., 2008).

At each developmental stage, there are certain tasks that children need to master to prepare them for the next stage of development. Later skills are often dependent on the achievement of earlier skills in the same domain. For example, children must learn to sit before they can stand. Though many skills and abilities of infants and small children go through this predictable sequence, it is known that they can do so at different rates and that qualitative differences can occur. These unstable developmental changes make the measurement of young children unique compared with that for older children (Bedford et al., 2013). Some skills are achieved at a predictable age, such as smiling by 8 weeks, while others vary in timescale, sometimes widely, such as walking, which is said to occur between 10 and 18 months. Sometimes, developmental variation can occur such as late walking or late talking, which may be familial. Some conditions can lead to developmental delay but are correctable, such as failure to thrive, hypothyroidism, or social isolation.

Check Your Progress

Factors to consider which influence early child development

Innate factors

- Genetic make-up
- Prenatal environment
- Temperament
- Basic safety
- Education
- Family support

Environmental factors

- Nutrition
- Housing
- Medical care

Thus early infant and child development is known to be rapid, dynamic, interactive, and variable. It is both universal and unique. Griffiths III helps the clinician to capture the unique developmental progression of each child across domains or avenues of learning, while at the same time acknowledging their individual background and culture.

Check Your Progress

- Remember there is an interplay of universal and unique factors that shape each child's individual development.
- Many cultural and environmental influences along with innate factors affect a child's development. Think about the different ways they can have an impact.
- A clinician needs to be aware of all of the influences that can impact development, as they carry out a developmental assessment.

Authentic Assessment of Children

The rapidly shifting nature of a child's early development poses problems for gaining an authentic assessment of their strengths, needs, and overall development. Early assessment and early intervention are considered crucial for growth and development, because experiences during early childhood can influence outcomes across the entire course of an individual's life (United Nations, 2010; WHO, 2007). Assessment has been defined by Snow and Van Hemel (2008), in their book *Early Childhood Assessment: Why, What, and How,* as the gathering of information on a child's background and their current skills, and using that information to help the child develop further within the context of the family, caregiving, and learning environments. Assessment, of course, is not an end in itself. Its goals are to obtain useful and accurate information about a child's skills, functioning, and environment to assist parents, health care providers, early educationalists, and others to better understand, plan for, and support the development and inclusion of a child with a disability (WHO, 2012).

Theories and new practices regarding developmental assessment continue to emerge. These include the use of qualitative and quantitative information, cultural sensitivity, and multidimensional approaches, as well as authentic and functional assessments. The focus of many of the proposed models of assessment, such as dynamic assessment and authentic assessment, is on meaningful application using real-life tasks and a focus on interaction and intervention. Therefore, it is essential to include both objective and subjective information about a child when conducting a comprehensive assessment. A key component of clinical assessment is measurement that can combine the use of quantitative and qualitative approaches to provide a better understanding of the child (Creswell & Plano Clark, 2018). Objectively, standardized developmental assessments provide valuable information by measuring functional abilities in children and identifying any deviations from the norm.

Parent and Professional Reports

Direct contacts with parents and other people familiar with the child are important starting points for better understanding and anticipating the needs of children with disabilities, and their families. Assessments are always more authentic when information is gathered from multiple perspectives and especially with naturalistic information from the various everyday settings of the child. The British Psychological Society (2011) recommends that clinicians always formulate from a broad-based, integrated, and multimodel perspective that locates personal meaning within its wider systemic, organizational, and societal contexts.

A comprehensive, authentic assessment will include working with parents and caregivers, gaining information from home and early education settings, and looking at the child's coping skills and behavior, as well as the important assessment of their neurodevelopmental milestones. This is why Griffiths III stresses that the voices of those most familiar with the child must be central to the process, because the goal of an early developmental assessment is to gain the most accurate picture of a child's development and capacities.

Observation of Child and Context

Griffiths III ensures that subjective information is gathered directly from the parent or caregiver and others, but also by engagement with the child. As part of a comprehensive assessment, direct observation and engagement with the child are both considered essential components. Positive engagement is also considered key to developmental gains (American Psychological Association, 2018), and the focus on engagement and connection using the developmental tasks in Griffiths III helps to target a child's functional abilities beyond the assessment process.

Challenges in the assessment of children have been reported because a child's development is dynamic in nature, and developmental domains are individually complex and interrelated. Development tends not to occur in a linear fashion, and in the younger child it slips in and out of "normality." For the first few years of life, the developmental domains are interconnected, and the major transitions in development occur in a dynamic interaction among the child, the social environment, and the context.

In a clinic setting, it is important to focus on the individual child in context. Factors known to affect a child's performance on testing include hunger, tiredness, or being in a strange place. Therefore, it must be remembered that a single test administered at a particular age provides only a snapshot of a child's abilities (Bedford et al., 2013). Griffiths III uses a range of test items and tasks that provide samples of, and a measure of, everyday behaviors in the child being assessed.

Research into the appropriateness of using the Griffiths Scales in different countries has revealed the need for adaptations of some tasks, translations of the instructions, and for country-specific normative information to be gathered. Studies have shown that the Griffiths Scales provide valuable diagnostic information about a range of developmental disorders in a wide variety of contexts across various countries. In order for a culturally appropriate standardized test such as Griffiths III to be used and available in contexts other than for the one for which it was developed, the solution appears to lie not in developing an indigenous test but rather in the adaptation of the measure. Creativity, ingenuity, and knowledge of the behavioral criteria associated with a construct in a specific culture are required when adapting test content or test tasks.

Check Your Progress

- Developmental assessments need to be authentic and relevant to understand, plan for, and support the development and inclusion of a child in everyday contexts.
- It is essential to include both objective and subjective information from multiple perspectives, especially from those who are most familiar with the child, when conducting a comprehensive assessment.
- In a clinical setting, focus on engaging directly with the child and their presentation on the day.
- Be aware of, and sensitive to, family differences in culture which may affect child-rearing practices and attitudes to illness and disability.

Understanding Griffiths III: The Test

One of the most important considerations for any developmental assessment is that the purpose in carrying out the assessment must be the primary focus to guide assessment decisions. Once the purpose is identified, the clinician chooses an appropriate assessment tool or measure to enable the child to show their unique and individual pattern of skills across a range of developmental domains. Standardized developmental tests have been viewed as the gold standard for outcome assessment, providing an objective, valid, and reliable evaluation of a child's development in comparison with the norm, and typically they provide standardized scores that can be used to classify developmental level (Mazer et al., 2012). Assessment measures with strong contextual validity and reliability allow us to better understand children's development and needs, which in turn allows for the design of more effective interventions.

Check Your Progress

- Before the assessment, identify the purpose and only then decide on your assessment tools.
- It is important to understand the psychometric properties of the assessment measures you use, including the validity and reliability of the test as well as any limitations to its use.

Item Gradients

Bracken (2004) defines *item gradients* as "how steeply graded standard scores are arranged in relation to their respective raw scores" (p. 41). This indicates how much difference a single test raw score can make to the normative interpretation of a child's test performance, and whether a difference in age of 1 month would seriously affect the item gradient. While a gentle gradient would be ideal, this is not always feasible, as it requires more test items to achieve. Bracken states further that tests for preschool children are notorious for having steep item gradients that allow only for a rough estimate of children's performance, but this is to be expected given the limited number of items. For Griffiths III, over 75% of the item gradients are within acceptable limits within month groups, while over 98% of gradients for adjoining months meet the expected standard of no more than one standard deviation difference. What this means in practice is that the test and norm tables provide sufficiently gentle item gradients to accurately determine the ability levels of a child, while being sensitive enough to highlight a child's relative areas of strength or weakness.

Check Your Progress

- Item gradients reflect how steeply graded standard scores are compared with their raw scores.
- Griffiths III item gradients can accurately determine the child's ability level, while also being able to identify the areas of strength or weakness.

Psychometric Strengths

The child's performance is analyzed in comparison with the normed group, which was the original Griffiths III standardization sample of children. The norms are interpreted using the normal distribution curve as a guide. Within the normal distribution, the clinician uses the norms to calculate how the child's performance compares with the typically developing sample. Figure 2.1 shows the interrelationships of normative scoring when using Griffiths III.

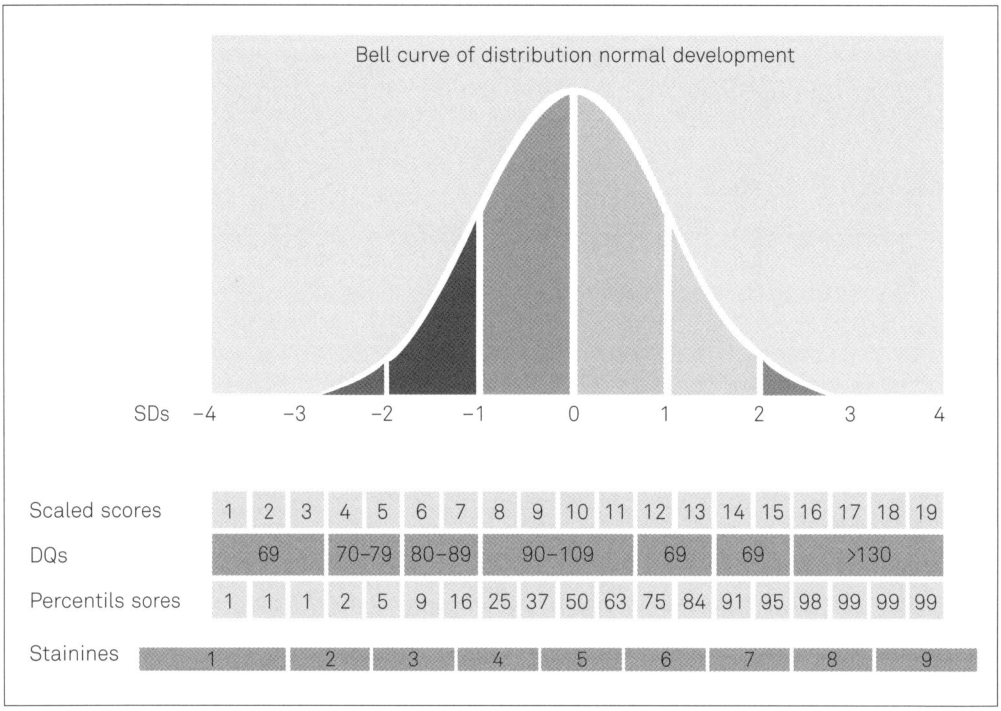

Figure 2.1. The interrelationships of normative scoring of Griffiths III

Norm-Referenced Scores

The following scores refer to Figure 2.1 (above) when using Griffiths III:

- Scaled scores (SS) have an average score of 10, with a range of 8–12.
- Development quotient (DQ) scores follow the normal curve with an average score between 90 and 109.
- Percentiles typically range from 1% to 99%, with an average of 50%. The percentile child's score refers to the percentage of same age peers who would be expected to score at or below the DQ score.

- Stanine test scores on a 9-point scale with an average of 5 and an *SD* of 2. A score of 9 indicates above average ability, and a score of 1 indicates very low relative achievement.
- A 95% confidence interval is the range in which, with 95% level of confidence, the achieved score would be expected to fall on any given day.

Developmental age equivalents are often used within the range of a normative test and represent the mean age that a particular raw score was achieved by that particular test's standardization sample, rather than accurate information about the child being assessed. Standard scores follow an equal-interval scale, but age equivalent raw scores are ordinal and do not increase at a constant rate from year to year, but with a flattening of the curve as age increases. Though they are not considered best practice, age equivalent scores do have some practical use. They can be useful when providing information to teachers or parents, to secure funding, to report scores when norms do not apply, and as a gross or initial measure to evaluate the severity of disorders and to guide additional testing (International Test Commission, 2001).

Check Your Progress

- Griffiths III norms are interpreted using the normal distribution curve as a guide when comparing the child's performance with the standardization sample.
- The norm-referenced scores in Griffiths III are standard scores, development quotients, percentiles, stanines, and confidence intervals.
- Developmental age equivalents are not normed scores but are derived from raw scores and should be used with caution.

Extremes (Upper and Lower Ends) of the Normal Curve of Developmental Skills

When the role of a test of general development is to identify deviation from the norm, as in Griffiths III, this can mean a loss of specificity and sensitivity for performances that fall at both ends of the distribution curve. The sparse comparison data from typically developing children at the lower end of the curve mean that for the 2.5% of children whose performance falls on the lower tail of the curve when compared against a norm group of typically developing children, the specific degree of impairment cannot be determined with any degree of confidence. So, for children whose development falls near or below the test floor, the test can confirm the level of disability, but the psychometric scores are mostly unreliable or lacking in meaning.

Researchers including Shapiro and colleagues (2008) have agreed that children who score at the floor of a normed test generally display a flat profile of standard scores of 1 or 0. Also that these standard scores do not sensitively report the true status of functioning in this cohort of children, hiding their individual strengths and weaknesses. It must be remembered then that standardized and normative scores constitute only one component of understanding a child's range of developing cognitive and developmental abilities.

Griffiths III when used with information such as background history, clinical observations, parental reports, and other sources of qualitative and quantitative information can provide an assessment framework for profiling the individual unique strengths and needs of children who fall outside of the boundaries of the test – that is, children who are over 6 years and/or whose performance falls below the floor of the test.

Check Your Progress

- A lack of specificity at the upper and lower ends of the distribution curve means that psychometric scores are unreliable.
- Scores near the floor of the test can confirm the level of disability but are not sensitive enough to identify strengths and weaknesses.

Subscale Significant Differences and Base Rates

When interpreting a child's assessed performance, some differences or variation across subscales would be expected. It is important to *interrogate the data* to discover whether such differences fall within the normal variation in child development, and whether the differences between subscale scores are statistically significant and if so, whether they indicate a significant strength or weakness (or delay) in the child's development.

It is also important for the clinician to know when it is optimal or not to report the *general development quotient* (GDQ) as an indicator of a child's overall performance. To check for significance, the clinician needs to calculate the difference between the child's highest and lowest subscale *standard scores* (SS) across the five subscales. The clinician should then look up the magnitude of the difference and the percentage of children who exhibit that difference. Generally, if the value of the scatter percentile (base rate) falls below the 10th to 15th percentile (Kaufman, 1976; Sattler, 1982), it is considered that the GDQ is not sufficient to represent the overall development of the child.

Table 2.1 provides a quick reference for interscale scatter. The base rates are indicated by the frequency or the percentage of children who obtained the range of scatter in the standardization sample. The significance of those scores that are considered significant is marked by the base rates within the shaded area, meaning a scatter of 8 points or more. Clinicians will use their professional judgment as to what they may consider significant. The magnitude of a scatter > 14 has not been included, because those base rates all occur in 0.0% of the population sample. The base rates within the shaded area suggest that the magnitude of the scatter indicates that it may not add value to use general development performance when describing the child's abilities, because the spread of scale scores between the five subscales (A to E) is too large.

Table 2.1. Base rates of interscale scatter by age bands

Scatter	Birth to 2 years 11 months (*n* = 232)	3 years to 5 years 11 months (*n* = 194)	Percentage of differences for the total cohort (*n* = 426)
14	0	0	0
13	0	1	0.5
12	0	2.6	1.2
11	0.4	2.6	1.4
10	2.2	2.6	2.3
9	4.7	4.1	4.5
8	10.3	8.2	9.4
7	18.5	15.5	17.1
6	29.3	29.4	29.3
5	48.7	50	49.3
4	68.1	73.2	70.4
3	88.8	86.1	87.6
2	97.8	96.9	97.4
1	99.1	99.9	99.1
0	100	100	100
Mean	4.7	4.7	4.7
Standard deviation	2.0	2.2	2.1

Check Your Progress

- When analyzing a child's scores, it is important to know if differences between subscale scores are statistically significant, and if so, whether that indicates a significant strength or weakness (or delay) in the child's development.
- Calculate the difference between the highest and lowest subscale standard scores across the five subscales: Look at Table 2.1 to check the magnitude of the difference and the percentage of children who exhibit that difference. If the magnitude of difference falls below the 10th to 15th percentiles, the GDQ should not be quoted.

Constructs and Subconstructs

The individual test items in Griffiths III can be viewed as general problem-solving processes measuring an underlying construct. A *construct* is said to be a skill or ability that is based on one or more established theories. The given construct cannot be measured directly, but it can be assessed using the child's performance on the test items, which have been devised to assess that construct.

Griffiths III was developed so that each domain and its constructs and subconstructs could be explored separately. Each developmental domain has a strong and unique identity which is made up of subconstructs which are operationalized to tap into sample behaviors chosen to assess, observe, and measure those concepts. It is these subconstructs that are considered valuable in the assessment of children with significant delays and disabilities.

In Griffiths III, test items measuring a single construct are sequentially placed from the developmental perspective, to help clinicians estimate the level that a particular child may be functioning at in that particular skill or ability. The constructs and subconstructs for each of the subscales are listed as follows:

Subscale A

The underlying constructs in Subscale A, foundations of learning, include critical aspects of cognition and learning that lay the foundation for later learning and education. These include a child's skills for learning, such as their attention, processing speed, and executive functions; their ways of thinking, such as reasoning, organizing, and planning; and memory and play. All of the test items fall under these constructs.

Subscale B

A child's overall language development is assessed in Subscale B, language and communication, and includes the use of language (expressive language) as well as the understanding of language (receptive language). It measures the progression from prelinguistic communicative intent, to the understanding and use of single words, to using two-word sentences, and on to the understanding and use of complex grammar. Aspects of cognition such as attention, listening, and verbal memory are also tapped into.

Subscale C

The constructs measured by the test items in Subscale C, eye and hand coordination, include the development of early visual perception, grasp, and object manipulation, as well as bilateral coordination, motor planning, visuomotor integration, graphomotor skills, and speed of movement and strength.

Subscale D

Under the main personal-social-emotional construct of Subscale D, subconstructs include a child's developing independence in activities of daily living and self-awareness, and their interpersonal and social skills, as well as the development of emotional understanding and expression, regulation, moral reasoning and perspective taking, and theory of mind.

Subscale E

The underlying constructs measured by the items in Subscale E, gross motor, include postural control, and gross motor and visual-spatial coordination. Later items measure balance, power, and strength.

Much information can be derived about the child's abilities by looking at their performance within each of the individual subscales. By noting the pattern of items passed and failed, and by checking to see what those items measure, specific strengths and needs can be pinpointed in each child's developmental profile. As the items are arranged in order of developmental difficulty, analysis of the items and underlying constructs can indicate areas to target for intervention. As an example, it could be observed that in Subscale B, a child may pass items that measure the underlying construct of receptive language, up to their age-expected level, but they may be unable to pass age-appropriate items that measure expressive language. Expressive language would then be an area to target for intervention. In Subscale D, the child may pass all the personal items related to the underlying subconstruct of independence in self-care but have difficulty passing some of the social or emotional items. Those specific failed items can then be analyzed and broadened, which would lead to intervention in the most appropriate areas of need.

Check Your Progress

- Each of the five subscales has a strong identity and is made up of underlying construct and subconstructs which have been operationalized to measure that concept.
- The subscales are foundations of learning, language and communication, eye and hand coordination, personal-social-emotional, and gross motor skills.
- Test items measuring a single construct are sequentially and developmentally placed, which can help estimate the level the child is functioning at in that skill.
- Check the pattern of items passed and failed, and note what constructs those items measure. This provides information about specific strengths and needs.

Data Aggregation and Disaggregation

In a normed test, individual test item data are aggregated by statistical analyses to produce scaled scores in relation to the standardization population. There is a loss of specificity and sensitivity for performances that fall at both ends of the distribution curve, so that if a child tests near or below the floor of the test, their scores lack detail (Pezzuti et al., 2018). According to Abualghaib and colleagues (2019), approximately 15% of the population lives with a disability, and 80% of those disabled individuals are in lower socioeconomic contexts. As normed tests compare the individual with their age or gender peers, such comparisons may stop at only placing their performance at a severely low level.

For a developmental test, such data aggregation would mean a failure in the fundamental assessment expectation, which is for the test to aid the clinician in describing the specific development of the child, including their relative areas of strength and weakness, and what the child is able to do and not to do. For those with disabilities, an assessment that only compares their performance relative to others, while not looking at the finer detail to understand the task performance, may compound the challenges they already face in accessing opportunities in mainstream society.

There is increasing recognition in the disability field that disaggregation of statistical scores may help to give further information on scores which fall in or below the tail of the normal curve (Abualghaib et al., 2019). In Griffiths III, it is possible to examine disaggregated test data through the use of the Griffiths III Quartile Charts. These enable comparison of the child's performance on each item, by age group and relative difficulty of the item. This allows the clinician to build a more comprehensive profile of the domains where the child is performing better or not, and to recommend a tailored support program for the child that uses their relative areas of strength as a scaffold to intervene in those areas of weakness.

The Quartile Charts

The Association for Research in Infant and Child Development (ARICD) has developed quartile charts that look at the level of difficulty of each individual subscale item. Use of the charts for fine-grained analysis of both items and constructs at the item level provides valuable information to the clinician in interpreting a child's performance on Griffiths III. The charts show all of the test items as they are presented in the year bands in the Griffiths III Record Book.

The quartile charts do not represent a calculated numerical value but present the percentage difficulty of the items in quartile groupings for each year. In each year band, the items grouped in Quartile 1 are the easiest items, and these items would be completed by 76–100% of typically developing children of that age year. Quartiles 2 and 3 contain items falling within the mid-range (26–75%) for that year. In Quartile 2, 51–75% of typically developing children achieve these items, and in Quartile 3, 26–50% typically developing children successfully achieve those items in the year. The items grouped in Quartile 4 are the hardest items in that year and were only completed by 1–25% of the typically developing children.

It is acknowledged that comparisons between typical developing children and those who have neurodevelopmental difficulties have many limitations. The quartile charts can assist clinicians in making clinical estimates of a child's level of functioning. When the charts are used to assist the qualitative developmental assessment of a child who would, in the examiner's opinion, meet the parameters of the standardized test, clinical judgment may be used, and if thought appropriate, the child may be said to be functioning at that particular developmental range of months.

Check Your Progress

- Data disaggregation helps analyze a child's performance beyond comparing their overall performance relative to others.
- The quartile charts were developed to allow for analysis of a child's performance at item level to help identify specific strengths and needs in their profile.

Key Concepts in Chapter 2

- The interplay of what is universal and unique in every child, and the nature of variation and culture
- Authentic assessment including
  - Reports from family and other professionals and
  - Observation of child and context
- Knowing the test – the test properties of Griffiths III:
  - Psychometric strengths,
  - Item gradients,
  - The extremes (upper and lower ends) of the normal curve of developmental skills,
  - Subscale significant differences and base rates,
  - The five subscales – constructs/subconstructs, and
  - Data aggregation/disaggregation

Discussion Questions

Personal Development

- Do I have enough knowledge of typical and atypical child development to carry out a comprehensive assessment?
- Can I remain flexible and observant while carrying out the assessment?

Psychoeducation

- Always remember to ask, What is the purpose of the assessment? and What referral question I am trying to answer?
- What assessment tool should I use? Would another test be more suitable?
- How will this assessment tool help or not help?

- Do the child's scores allow for reporting of their GDQ?
- Does advanced ability in one area mask a difficulty in another?
- Have I checked in with the parents or caregivers? Are adult expectations consistent with a child's capabilities?

Advocacy

Development is a complex concept that is dependent on multiple factors from both inside and outside the child. Remember the exactly "average child" is a statistical creation that very rarely exists; more typically, any child will present with fluctuating patterns of peaks and troughs across developmental areas and time. Most children will fall within the broad average range in each area.

References

Abualghaib, O., Groce, N. E., Simeu, N., Carew, M. T., & Mont, D. (2019). Making visible the invisible: Why disability-disaggregated data is vital to "leave no-one behind." *Sustainability, 11,* 3091. https://doi.org/10.3390/su11113091

American Psychological Association. (2018). *Guidelines for assessment and intervention with people with disabilities.* https://www.apa.org/pi/disability/resources/assessment-disabilities.aspx

Bedford, H., Walton, S., & Ahn, J. (2013). *Measures of child development: A review.* UCL Institute of Child Health.

Bracken, B. A. (2004). *Psychoeducational assessment of preschool children* (3rd ed.). Lawrence Erlbaum.

British Psychological Society. (2011). *Good practice guidelines on the use of psychological formulation.*

Creswell, J. W., & Plano Clark, V. L. (2018). *Designing and conducting mixed methods research.* Sage.

Ertem, I. O., Krishnamurthy, V., Mulaudzi, M. C., Sguassero, Y., Balta, H., Gulumser, O., Bilik, B., Srinivasan, R., Johnson, B., Gan, G., Calvocoressi, L., Shabanova, V., & Forsyth, B. W. C. (2018). Similarities and differences in child development from birth to age 3 years by sex and across four countries: A cross-sectional, observational study. *Lancet Global Health, 6*(3), 279–291. https://doi.org/10.1016/S2214-109X(18)30003-2

International Test Commission, (2001). International guidelines for test use. *International Journal of Testing, 1*(2), 93–114.

Kaufman, A. S. (1976). A new approach to the interpretation of the test scatter on the WISC-R. *Journal of Learning Disabilities, 9,* 160–168. https://doi.org/10.1177/002221947600900308

Knickmeyer, R. C., Knickmeyer, R. C., Gouttard, S., Kang, C., Evans, D., Wilber, K., Smith, J. K., Hamer, R. M., Lin, W., Gerig, G., & Gilmore, J. H. (2008). A structural MRI study of human brain development from birth to 2 years. *Journal of Neuroscience, 28,* 12176–12182. https://doi.org/10.1523/JNEUROSCI.3479-08.2008

Maschinot, B. (2008). *The changing face of the United States: The influence of culture on child development.* ZERO TO THREE.

Mazer, B., Majnemer, A., Dahan-Oliel, N., & Sebestyen, I. (2012). Global developmental assessments. In Majnemer A. (Ed.), *Clinical and research measures for children with developmental disability: Framed by the ICF-CY.* MacKeith Press

Pezzuti, L., Nacinovich, R., Oggiano, S., Bomba, M., Ferri, R., La Stella, A., Rossetti, S., & Orsini, A. (2018). Beyond the floor effect on the WISC-IV in individuals with Down syndrome: Are there cognitive strengths and weaknesses? *Journal of Intellectual Disability Research*, 62(7), 593–603. https://doi.org/10.1111/jir.12499

Sattler, J. M. (1982). *Assessment of children's intelligence and special abilities* (2nd ed.). Allyn & Bacon.

Shapiro, E. G., Whitley, C. B., & Eisengart, J. B. (2018). Beneath the floor: Re-analysis of neurodevelopmental outcomes in untreated Hurler syndrome. *Orphanet Journal of Rare Diseases, 13,* 1–8. https://doi.org/10.1186/s13023-018-0817-3

Snow, C. E., & Van Hemel, S. B. (Eds.). (2008). *Early childhood assessment: Why, what, and how.* National Academy Press.

United Nations. (2010). *Status of the convention on the rights of the child: Report of the secretary-general.* Sixty-fifth General Assembly of the United Nations, New York, August 2, 2010.

Villar, J., Fernandes, M., Purwar, M., Staines-Urias, E., Di Nicola, P., Cheikh Ismail, L., Ochieng, R., Barros, F., Albernaz, E., Victora, C., Kunnawar, N., Temple, S., Giuliani, F., Sandells, T., Carvalho, M., Ohuma, E., Jaffer, Y., Noble, A., Gravett, M., ... & Kennedy, S. (2019). Neurodevelopmental milestones and associated behaviours are similar among healthy children across diverse geographical locations. *Nature Communications, 10*(1), 511. https://doi.org/10.1038/s41467-018-07983-4

World Health Organization. (2007). *Early childhood development: A powerful equalizer.* https://www.who.int/social_determinants/resources/ecd_kn_report_07_2007.pdf

World Health Organization. (2012). *Early childhood development and disability: Discussion paper.* https://apps.who.int/iris/handle/10665/75355

Chapter 3

Using Griffiths III to Interpret, Plan, and Report a Child's Needs

Hilary Lane and Johan Cronje

This chapter describes using Griffiths III to interpret and describe a child's performance in order to better formulate the case and provide feedback and recommendations. It considers the fact that a developmental assessment must use all of the available information about the child from a range of sources – subjective and objective, formal and informal – to capture the essence of each child's competencies. Only by interpreting and analyzing the results at their different levels of information can the clinician formulate a comprehensive picture and provide recommendations to ensure the child reaches their fullest potential. Blanton and Jaccard (2006) consider that awareness of psychometric limitations is of value and that "a researcher who appreciates the gap between a psychological metric and a psychological reality knows to look past a person's score and search for something meaningful" (p. 39). Wilcox and Schroeder (2015) have noted that this process of evaluation involves the meaningful synthesis or merging of different kinds of results (scored results and individual perceptions of received information), and Aylward (2009) has discussed qualitative information combined with quantitative data in developmental testing. Early identification of developmental issues can make a significant difference for infants and young children experiencing developmental delays or disabilities.

Clinicians are generally aware that many considerations need to be addressed when assessing a child with atypical development. The British Psychological Society (BPS), the American Psychological Association (APA), and the International Test Commission (ITC) all offer guidance and recommendations for the assessment and intervention of people with disabilities.

Check Your Progress

- A clinician needs to gather all available information from a range of familiar sources before interpreting and formulating their hypotheses.
- The clinician often needs to look beyond the achieved scores to find what is meaningful.
- Follow your professional body's guidance and recommendations when assessing children with atypical development.

Administration and Scoring of Griffiths III

Griffiths III is intended for use by professionals qualified in its administration and interpretation through training, education, and experience. It is a *closed test*, meaning that it is only available to pediatricians, psychologists, and certain other allied health professionals who undergo approved training before becoming registered in its use.

To ensure that the clinician can make correct and proper inferences, it is essential that the assessment be conducted in the standardized format as laid out in the *Griffiths III: Griffiths Scales of Child Development, 3rd Edition. Part II: Administration and Scoring* (Green et al., 2016).

Clinicians need to adhere to the following:

- Use of a new Griffiths III record and drawing book for each child,
- Strict adherence to test administration instructions,
- Correct calculation of chronological age and rounded age, and
- Use of correct basal and ceiling points. Administering and scoring the test in a specified standardized format provides for objectivity and reduces subjectivity in testing. Clinicians should be aware of whether they have a particular bias when scoring individual items, in that they can often underestimate or overestimate a child's abilities and so give credit, or not, owing to their own personal bias or preconceived ideas.

Once the face-to-face assessment is complete, the clinician should ensure that:

- Meticulous attention must be paid to the calculation of the three raw scores: (1) the Year Raw Score, (2) the Subscale Raw Score, and (3) the General Development Raw Score.
- The raw score subscale summary section should be recorded on the front cover of the record book.
- The raw data should then be transferred to the analysis sheet on the inside of the back cover of the record book.

Using the *Griffiths III: Griffiths Scales of Child Development, 3rd Edition. Part III: Norms* (Foxcroft et al., 2016), the clinician converts the raw scores to norm-referenced scores. The norm-referenced scores include the scaled scores, development quotients, percentiles, stanines, and confidence intervals for the inherent error of measurement. Each subscale is scored separately, giving a separate level of functioning in the specific domain. This allows for comparison across the five developmental areas. The *general development quotient* (also referred to simply as the GDQ) indicates the overall level of functioning.

It is known that norming standardization can convey important and useful information about relative standing but cannot convey absolute standing (Visser et al., 2012). It must be remembered that a young child's performance is variable and is influenced by several factors, so great care must be taken in drawing inferences from the statistical data. A number of personal and external variables on the day can add to the complexity of assessing a child, especially those with atypical needs. The compounding factor of disability leads to a multifaceted conundrum, especially when examining a measure or test which is standardized against a sample of typically developing children. Nevertheless, these measures remain part of the assessment process to provide information about the child's developmental capacity.

Griffiths III can be used directly with the child to obtain both objective quantitative and qualitative information across the range of developmental domains or avenues of learning. Although developmental domains are considered individually, the experienced clinician will always consider how one particular domain relates to other areas of development.

Check Your Progress

- When conducting an assessment, use a new record book, adhere strictly to the administration guidelines, remember to calculate the child's rounded age, and use basal and ceiling scores.
- Calculate each year's raw score, each subscale's raw score, and the general development raw score.
- Using the raw scores, under the child's chronological age, the norm tables provide scaled scores, development quotients, developmental age equivalents, percentiles, stanines, and confidence intervals for each of the subscales as well as norms for general or overall development.

What to Do When Comparative Statistics Are Inappropriate

Visser and colleagues (2012) have noted that standardized instruments can only be used for children with special needs if such children undergo a developmental process that is only quantitatively, and not qualitatively, different from that of typically developing children. In developmental tests, an ordinal development of skills is assumed, however, Levy (2018) noted that the hallmarks of developmental disorders are disrupted developmental timing and slow acquisitional pace.

In their standardized and normative format, standardized assessment measures are generally not appropriate to use with children with significant developmental needs. Standardized metrics have clearly defined issues in relation to children with developmental disability. Ratio development quotients reflect the rate of development and are not comparable at different age levels because the standard deviation (variance) of the ratios does not remain constant. Also, confidence intervals vary considerably. So comparative statistics are inappropriate, and attempting to use scores is not advised.

In general, clinicians want to extract more meaningful information about a particular child, rather than just a general confirmation of disability, though that might be necessary also. Individualization is central to the design and development of intervention plans for children with disabilities, so considerable experience in working with children with significant delays and disabilities is advised and necessary. This can provide knowledge about the functional characteristics of a particular disability which could determine whether or not the disability is related to the construct being measured. This ensures correct interpretation of assessment.

Check Your Progress

- Be aware of the limitations of standardized tests when used with children with significant developmental delays and disabilities.
- Remember a child's diagnosis may impact their development in many different ways, so neurodevelopmental knowledge and experience is essential in interpreting their assessments.

Accommodations and Modifications Using Griffiths III

Accommodations

Griffiths III, though standardized in its administration when used in a normative format, allows for certain accommodations when the clinician considers it necessary. Accommodations are test adaptations that allow the child to demonstrate what they know without changing the target skill being measured in the test situation. Accommodations do not change the content of instruction, or give the child an unfair advantage, or change the skills or knowledge that a test measures. They do not reduce performance expectations, as the purpose is to ensure equal access. With accommodations, the child does the same test, but their individual needs are accommodated, it is the *how* that is changed.

In the Griffiths III various accommodations in testing can be made once the explicit instructions for standardized testing are adhered to – that is, *instruction accommodations* could be verbal repetition of instructions where allowed. Often the parent or caregiver can be asked to assist with testing, guided by the tester and again only by asking the correct instruction. Though it is recommended to complete each of the subscales fully and in order, if possible, the tester must remain flexible, and the order of administering subscales or test items may be changed. *Response accommodations* include allowing the child to point or indicate their response by whatever means they can – for example, finger pointing, eye pointing, etc. The child may need a number of sessions to complete the test or require frequent breaks during the sessions.

Modifications

Modifications, on the other hand, are test adaptations that allow the child to demonstrate what they can do, but the target skill is reduced in some way. Modifications usually lessen the complexity of the tasks required. If the validity of a test item or the content of instruction is affected or altered, the change is a modification – not an accommodation. With modifications, the test items themselves are modified – the *what* is changed. The International Test Commission (2001) has noted that considerable care and expertise is needed when the mode of a test has to be changed to accommodate the needs of people with disabilities. It also notes that given a lack of information about people with disabilities on tests, it is often more appropriate for test results to be used in a qualitative manner.

When using Griffiths III, an experienced clinician will tailor accommodations and modifications to the individual child, and the test items can provide a structure for looking at the strengths and needs of the child within the framework of the test. By using the Vygotskian (Vygotsky, 1978) principles of zones of proximal development, scaffolding, and the social context of learning, a tester can perform an analysis of the individual test items *relative* to what the child can do with and without help. The difference between the child's higher level of potential and the lower level of actual development indicates the *zone of proximal development*. This dynamic form of assessment is an interactive approach that embeds intervention within the assessment procedure.

The zone of proximal development or testing of the limits can provide information about a child's learning potential as the focus of the assessment is on what the child knows, what the child can do, what skills are emerging, and what needs to be done to help the child's development based on this information. Such testing goes beyond the only responses allowed in the standardized format and allows for accommodations and modifications as required. Performance in one developmental domain does not necessarily equate with performance in the other domains, and there can be significant variations between domains. Intervention can then be targeted by starting where the child is at and in this way will facilitate progress further.

Check Your Progress

- Accommodations in the test are allowed, as long as the test itself is not changed in any way.
- Modifications change the actual test, so scores are rendered invalid.
- With an experienced clinician, test accommodations and modifications can be used in a dynamic manner to provide valuable information on the child's potential in all developmental domains.

Quartile Charts

When assessing a child with atypical development, the quartile charts can be used to examine the test items the child successfully completes, or is unable to complete, and to plot the quartile in which those items fall across the five subscales. To report the child's results, it can be stated that the individual test items achieved by the child were achieved by the typically developing children in the standardization sample within the listed quartile for that year band. Descriptions of skill achievement at specific item level can help the clinician define a child's strengths. The charts can also help to analyze which test items were not achieved. This is valuable information to assist with future intervention and educational planning.

Check Your Progress

- The quartile charts provide guidance when interpreting a child's performance in comparison with the standardization sample.
- The quartile charts indicate at what level the normative group successfully completed the skills within a 3-month range.
- Analysis using the quartile charts of the skills and the underlying constructs, which were achieved or not by the child, can provide specific areas for intervention and further support.

Case Formulation

Once all of the information is gathered from multiple sources and through direct informal and formal assessment measures, the clinician sets about integrating, interpreting, and analyzing the information to make a case formulation. This tells the *story* of the particular child being assessed. Analysis of all of the information gathered about the child generates various hypotheses in relation to the referral question. These hypotheses lead to the case formulation and plans for intervention. The information gathered across and within the Griffiths III subscales, along with qualitative clinical observations, such as the child's listening skills, attention, perseverance, enthusiasm, and imagination, together help the clinician formulate a clinical opinion of the child's level of skills and functional abilities and also form a descriptive, holistic profile of the child. Once the individual child's skill levels have been assessed through the use of Griffiths III, it is then imperative to use those levels to expand its functional aspects in the child's life. Confirmation with the parents that the observations and skills that have been observed are representative of what is seen at home and in other settings on a daily basis provides ecological validity for your results.

Check Your Progress

- The case formulation tells the story of the child by integrating and analyzing all available information.
- The case formulation generates a holistic, descriptive profile of the child's skills, abilities, and competencies, and indicates specific areas for intervention.
- The profile needs to be representative of the child's day-to-day functioning, as seen by the people most familiar with them.

Recommendations and Intervention

Once the assessment of the child is complete and the results collated, the formulation and interpretations made, recommendations in terms of objectives and desired outcomes should be made in conjunction with the parents. The next steps for learning are agreed based on the developmental performance of the child. Talk with the parents, teachers, and therapists about techniques that facilitate the child's learning. The clinician can use all of the qualitative information gained during the assessment, specifically how the child could successfully complete a range of tasks with help and guidance but not yet independently. These provide small steps that the child can learn to achieve with minimal assistance to promote their development.

Recommendations should be formulated in an optimistic manner, providing clear indications as to the construction of an appropriately challenging individual intervention program.

Check Your Progress

- Recommendations need to be clear, positive, and relevant, with a list of objectives and desired outcomes.
- Steps to help the child achieve the desired outcomes should be identified using all of the information gained during the assessment.

Assessment Feedback and the Griffiths III Report

Following an assessment, discussion of the findings with the parents or caregivers can be challenging, especially if a global developmental delay is found. Williams and Essex (2004) have noted that the term "delay" may be understood by the parents as the child having the ability to catch up, and this is often not the case. Feedback with parents and disclosure of ongoing developmental disabilities, whether delivered antenatally, postnatally, or in the early years needs to be delivered sensitively and empathetically. Parents report that a positive experience of the way information is communicated is helpful when faced with uncertainty.

A written developmental report is often the only permanent record of the assessment process; therefore, great care and consideration needs to be taken when writing the report. Providing verbal feedback on an assessment relies on the parent's or caregiver's understanding and memory and often cannot be revisited. The purpose of the report is to communicate the findings of the assessment. One needs to provide a comprehensive, respectful picture of the child, emphasizing strengths and positive elements, as well as stating challenges in performance. The report should always be prepared with the readers in mind. Remember that "A report may influence a child and family for years to come – drafting it deserves care and attention" (Green et al., 2016, p. 99).

Clinicians' written reports should follow the guidelines of their professional bodies and organizations. However, a framework or template for the written report is also outlined in the *Griffiths III: Griffiths Scales of Child Development, 3rd Edition. Part II: Administration and Scoring* (Green et al., 2016, pp. 99–100). It includes the following:

- Clarification of the referral question is usually the basis for the assessment process and should be at the beginning of your report.
- Background information relevant to the child should be summarized, which includes parent, carer, and/or family factors; medical and health history; environmental factors; and any previous assessments or examinations.
- List all the tests and measures used during the assessment. Qualify why a particular test such as Griffiths III was chosen. It is the clinician's responsibility to choose the most appropriate instrument for a particular child in a particular context.
- Clinical observations are important as they provide qualitative information directly from the child. The child's test behavior and presentation may be important factors when making the case formulation.
- In the next section are the test scores and results. Many clinicians like to use tables or figures for the scores and numerical findings. These may be helpful when the reader understands what they stand for; however, remember parents and others may not understand the numerical results.
- Always provide interpretation of the results provided. This can be done by including both factual descriptive statements and then interpretive statements of the results. Remember to adhere to descriptors, statistics, and other information contained in the Griffiths III manuals or resources provided by ARICD.
- Always remember current levels of functioning are only snapshots in time. Do not overgeneralize from limited data or make conclusions if test results are not definitive or are not backed up by other sources of data. Remember, skills that have not yet evolved clearly cannot be assessed until such time as they might reasonably be expected to be present.
- A summary section clarifies the main issue for the reader and is a process of synthesis for the writer.
- In the concluding section of the report, always provide practical, concrete, reasonable, and attainable goals, which should include advice on the next steps for therapy, intervention, and child and family support.

Collaboration with the parents and significant others in the child's life adds significant value and weight to the assessment. Respect the parent or caregiver's wishes and expectations and always build on their cultural and family strengths.

Check Your Progress

- Verbal feedback to parents or caregivers should be delivered in a clear, sensitive manner and free of jargon. Check their understanding and encourage questions.
- Provide evidence from your assessment for your conclusions and recommendations.
- A written report will be a permanent record, so great care and consideration needs to be taken when drafting it.
- Include all qualitative and quantitative information, with an interpretation and explanations of what all terms mean.
- The report summary and conclusions should synthesize the results of the assessment and lead to practical, attainable goals for the child and family.

Key Concepts in Chapter 3

- Administering scoring and interpreting the Griffiths III
- What to do when comparative statistics are inappropriate
- Adaptations and modifications
- Using the quartile charts
- Case formulation
- Recommendations and interventions
- Assessment feedback and the Griffiths III report

Discussion Questions

Personal Development

- Do I have a clear understanding of how to administer, score, and interpret Griffiths III?
- Do I have an understanding of how to use Griffiths III with children who score near or below the floor of the test?
- Do I know the test well enough to use it in a flexible manner to accommodate the needs of children with disabilities?

Psychoeducation

- Griffiths III helps to provide a comprehensive picture of a child's overall level of general development, and results in each of the subscales can identify strengths, needs, and areas for learning, across the developmental domains.
- Construct and subconstruct analysis will provide information on a child's underlying skills, which may impact on overall development and provide information for areas of further development.
- Griffiths III can be used as a framework for qualitative assessment to help determine an approximate level of functioning for children who score below the floor of the test.
- Always include and be aware of the needs of the family when carrying out a developmental assessment.

Advocacy

- Early assessment and intervention are considered essential to promote optimum outcomes.
- Griffiths III is a unique clinical instrument that enables an innovative assessment of the strengths, needs, skills, and abilities of children with a wide range of neurodevelopmental abilities and disabilities.

Quantitative Elements of Griffiths III Used in the Case Studies in Section III

- Normative scoring is used to achieve standard scores, development quotients, developmental age equivalents, percentiles, stanines, and confidence intervals.
- Base rate analysis is completed, and subscale significant differences are revealed.

Qualitative Elements of Griffiths III Used in the Case Studies in Section III

Qualitative elements of Griffiths III include its use

- As a framework for a qualitative assessment,
- For construct and subconstruct analysis, and
- To create quartile charts.

References

Aylward, G. P. (2009). Developmental screening and assessment: What are we thinking? *Journal of Developmental & Behavioral Pediatrics, 2009*, 30, 169–173. https://doi.org/10.1097/DBP.0b013e31819f1c3e

Blanton, H., & Jaccard, J. (2006). Arbitrary metrics in psychology. *American Psychologist, 61*, 27–41. https://doi.org/10.1037/0003-066X.61.1.27

Foxcroft, C., Stroud, L., et al. (2016). *Griffiths III: Griffiths scales of child development, 3rd edition. Part III: Norms.* Hogrefe.

Green, E., Stroud, L., O'Connell, R., Bloomfield, S., Cronje, J., Foxcroft, C., Hurter, K., Lane, H., Marais, R., Marx, C., McAlinden, P., Paradice, R., & Venter, D. (2016). *Griffiths III: Griffiths scales of child development, 3rd edition. Part II: Administration and scoring.* Hogrefe.

International Test Commission. (2001). International guidelines for test use. *International Journal of Testing, 1*(2), 93–114.

Levy, Y. (2018). Developmental delay reconsidered: The critical role of age-dependent, co- variant development. *Frontiers in Psychology, 9*, 1–10. https://doi.org/10.3389/fpsyg.2018.00503

Visser, L., Ruiter, S. A. J., van der Meulen, B. F., Ruijssenaars, W. A. J. J. M., & Timmerman, M. E. (2012). A review of standardized developmental assessment instruments for young children and their applicability for children with special needs. *Journal of Cognitive Education and Psychology, 11*, 102–127. https://doi.org/10.1891/1945-8959.11.2.102

Vygotsky, L. S. (1978). *Mind in society.* Harvard University Press.

Wilcox, G., & Schroeder, M. (2015). What comes before report writing? Attending to clinical reasoning and thinking errors in school psychology. *Journal of Psychoeducational Assessment, 33*, 652–661. https://doi.org/10.1177/0734282914562212

Williams, A., & Essex, C. (2004). Developmental delay or failure to arrive? *Developmental Medicine & Child Neurology, 46*(7), 502. https://doi.org/10.1017/s0012162204240828

Section III

Griffiths III Case Studies

Every child is a different kind of flower, and all together, make this world a beautiful garden.

– Tough Like Taylor

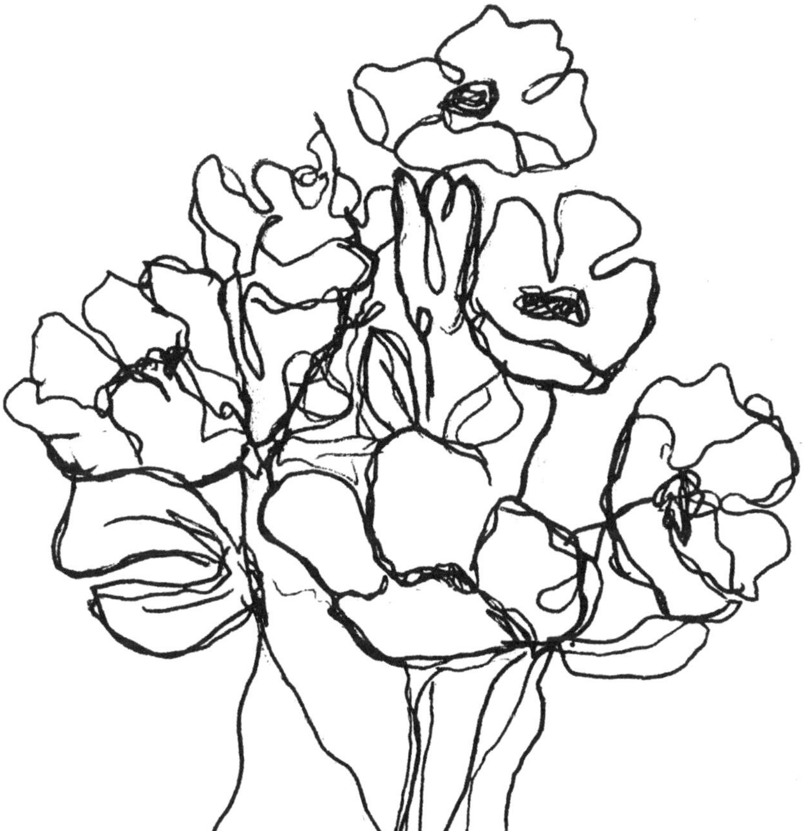

Zone 1: Children With Symptoms of Learning, Physical, or Sensing Difficulties	
Chapter 4	Divoc: School Readiness in a Child With Developmental Language Disorder
Chapter 5	Mary: Nonstandardized Use of Griffiths III as a Qualitative Assessment of a Child Over 6 Years
Chapter 6	Poppy: A Child With Hearing Impairment and Congenital Cytomegalovirus Infection
Zone 2: Children With Dominant Symptoms of the Autistic Spectrum	
Chapter 7	Hugo: A Brazilian Child Diagnosed With Autism Spectrum Disorder
Chapter 8	Jamie: Assessing a Child With High Functioning Autism
Chapter 9	Eli: Assessing a Child With Low Functioning Autism
Chapter 10	Victor: Resilience in the COVID-19 Pandemic
Zone 3: Children With Symptoms of General Developmental Delay	
Chapter 11	Johan: A Swedish Boy Who Fits the ESSENCE Description
Chapter 12	Sam: Neurodevelopmental Concerns in a Preterm Infant
Zone 4: Children With Syndromes or Genetic Disorders	
Chapter 13	Elena: Assessing a Child With Down Syndrome
Chapter 14	Ben: A Boy with a Mosaic Form of Chromosome 18q21.1 Deletion
Chapter 15	Milly: A Child With Fetal Alcohol Syndrome Disorder
Chapter 16	Ava: A Girl With Phenylketonuria and Typical Development
Zone 5: Children With Variability in Typical Development	
Chapter 17	Leo: A Child With Variability Above the Range of Typical Development
Chapter 18	James: A Child With Variability Within the Range of Typical Development

Zone 1

Zone 1: Children With Symptoms of Learning, Physical, or Sensing Difficulties	
Chapter 4	Divoc: School Readiness in a Child With Developmental Language Disorder
Chapter 5	Mary: Nonstandardized Use of Griffiths III as a Qualitative Assessment of a Child Over 6 Years
Chapter 6	Poppy: A Child With Hearing Impairment and Congenital Cytomegalovirus Infection

Chapter 4

Divoc: School Readiness in a Child With Developmental Language Disorder

Rosemary O'Connell

The Context

The author of this chapter is a retired psychologist who worked as both an educational psychologist and a clinical psychologist. This case study describes developmental assessment and decisions about school placement in a child diagnosed with a developmental language disorder. The child is a hypothetical case based on the author's 40 years of experience of assessing similar children with a range of developmental difficulties in Irish clinical and educational settings. The child in the study has moved home and country, now has only one parent, and has language difficulties. This chapter has the following purposes:

- To illustrate how a parent may make well-meaning decisions about school entry, based on "common sense" but insufficient information,
- To discuss the concept of school readiness, and
- To address the question of school choice where specialized provision is available.

The Child

Divoc, aged 5 years 6 months at the time of Griffiths III assessment, was seen in Ireland for assessment of need under the Disability Act 2005, at his preschool and at home. An only child, he was born in the Czech Republic to English-speaking parents. After a protracted labor and forceps delivery, he spent some time in a neonatal intensive care unit. He was sick a lot when he was a baby, with constant ear infections and asthma. He crawled at 10 months and walked at 13 months. First words started at about 12 months, but Divoc developed many words of his own which often bore no resemblance to the real word: for example, "bottle" was "schlaa," "Sherpa" (the cat) was "Dab."

Divoc and his mother moved to live in Ireland when he was 2 years 6 months old. His father had no further contact with them, and Divoc missed him, often calling for him at first. His mother thought his speech was a little behind for his age, but attributed this to the fact that he had not started in preschool, and to the several different house moves they had made after moving to Ireland, until they settled in a rural area some 10 km (6.2 miles) from the nearest small town. Divoc began in the local preschool aged 3 years 4 months, twice a week.

Following his speech and language evaluation (see below in The Condition), Divoc began attending weekly speech therapy and was placed on a waiting list to be considered for acceptance into a special class for children with language disorder the following school year when he would be 5 years 4 months old. No referrals (e.g., for psychological or developmental assessment) were made at this time.

From the September after his fourth birthday Divoc attended preschool daily. He made friends with one quiet little girl, but sometimes hit other children when he could not say what he wanted to say. His favorite activities were engines and robots, counting, and jigsaws. At the end of the academic year, a detailed report from his preschool group leader noted poor language skills and limited concentration, and refusal to take part in certain activities (including listening to a story in the group, singing songs). Divoc's speech and language had made some progress, but his social presentation was immature for his age. Unfortunately, his language needs were considered to be less urgent than those of other children on the waiting list for the Special Language Class, and he did not succeed in getting a place in the class. The Admissions Board for the Language Class recommended that he should be referred for psychological assessment. This referral was made by his GP, who was made aware of his language difficulties for the first time. The GP arranged a hearing test for Divoc, which showed that he had good hearing in both ears. The GP also arranged for Divoc to be seen by the local autism services, and diagnostic screening ruled out autism as a possible factor.

After consultation with the GP, his mother and preschool teacher decided to keep him a further year in preschool, even though he would be 6 years 4 months on school entry. It was considered that he was not ready for school. This decision was made on the basis of his language difficulties and immature behavior.

Check Your Progress

- Where and with whom does Divoc live?
- Why did he have this assessment?

The Condition

Divoc's language skills were of concern to his preschool staff. With his mother's consent, he was referred for speech and language assessment: The waiting list was 16 weeks, and he was seen when he was aged 4 years 2 months. On assessment of his speech and language skills, the therapist confirmed that Divoc's scores indicated that he had "moderately delayed receptive language, and mildly delayed expressive language skills. . . . Divoc presented with a disorder in his use and understanding of the semantic content of language. This presentation is consistent with a diagnosis of developmental language disorder" as specified in the *Diagnostic and Statistical Manual of Mental Disorders*, 5th edition (DSM-5 in American Psychiatric Association, 2013). The *International Classification of Diseases*, 11th edition (ICD-11; World Health Organisation, 2019), gives diagnostic criteria for this as

> Developmental language disorder is characterised by persistent deficits in the acquisition, understanding, production or use of language (spoken or signed), that arise during the developmental period, typically during early childhood, and cause significant limitations in the individual's ability to communicate. The individual's ability to understand, produce or use language is markedly below what would be expected given the individual's age. The language deficits are not explained by another neurodevelopmental disorder or a sensory impairment or neurological condition, including the effects of brain injury or infection.

The *International Classification of Diseases,* 10th edition (ICD-10; World Health Organization, 2016), also mentions that it may also be associated with broadly defined social-emotional behavioral disturbances.

Check Your Progress

- What did the speech and language assessment show?

The Consultation

Developmental assessment was requested to help with the formulation of a program to help Divoc make the transition from preschool to school. Assessment was commenced in preschool, with observations of Divoc in the group, both indoors and outdoors. He was aged 5 years 6 months. The observations confirmed the interpersonal social difficulties outlined by his preschool teacher. Formal individualized testing was started in the preschool resource room, but Divoc was resistant, and his concentration was so poor that testing was completed in his own home in a quiet room, in three sessions over 2 weeks. He was a very restless and somewhat anxious child, needing a high level of success and a higher intensity of adult praise and encouragement than should have been necessary for his age. Divoc's scores on the Griffiths III Scales of Child Development are shown in Table 4.1.

Table 4.1. Divoc's scores on Griffiths III

Subscale	Scaled score	Development quotient	Percentile	Stanine
Subscale A	12	109	71	6
Subscale B	3	59	1	1
Subscale C	8	90	27	4
Subscale D	0	50	< 1	1
Subscale E	10	100	49	5

The general development quotient was not used, because of the large variation between the scaled scores of the subtests. The Griffiths III base rate tables, which give the degree of significance of the spread of scores, showed six significant differences between the subscale pairings. These could generate much further discussion about the nature of Divoc's language difficulties and other aspects of his cognitive functioning, but are not the focus of this case study. The magnitude of the base rate scatter indicated that the general development quotient was not sufficient to represent Divoc's overall development.

Divoc's strengths are in the Griffiths Constructs of Ways of Thinking, Memory and practical problem-solving skills as measured by Subscale A. His physical balance, rhythm, gross body coordination, and strength, as measured by Subscale E, are also at a good level for his age. These strengths provide opportunities for success in his educational programs, and scaffolding with very slightly more difficult tasks will help develop these two areas further.

While he was quite good at construction tasks, and had the coordination to dress himself and to eat neatly without spilling at table, Divoc showed minor difficulties with graphomotor skills, in particular with pencil grip, and some problems with placement and spatial planning when drawing. This apparent discrepancy may be due to the fact that writing uses many 'association' brain areas, which link sensory input areas of the brain with motor output portions of the central nervous system. Dressing, undressing, and eating do not use many of these association areas, rather they use the main motor and coordination areas of the brain (Lyons, 2020).

Eye and hand coordination functioning was within average range for his age, but analysis of his functioning on Scale C indicated that Divoc's results on items measuring the constructs fine motor coordination, graphomotor, and bilateral coordination were less developed than those on tests of motor planning and construction.

The clinical and educational concerns remained focused on his language and social functioning. Griffiths III scores supported results from Divoc's speech and language assessment. His mother stated that language was the area of most concern to her and felt that Divoc would have difficulty in early primary school. Some improvement had been seen since speech therapy commenced, but Divoc continued to be very exasperated and frustrated by his inability to communicate effectively through language. Divoc's name remained on the list for possible admission to the Language Special class. In the meantime, speech therapy continued weekly with programs being carried out by his mother and his preschool.

The low results on the personal-social-emotional subscale of the Griffiths Scales indicated that a more detailed analysis of Subscale D scores would be useful to pinpoint areas of moral reasoning. The analysis proved very helpful as it ruled out difficulties in the self-help area. On the relevant items in Griffiths III, Divoc showed competence in utensil use at home and was reported to eat independently and efficiently at table. He was also able to dress and undress without difficulty. The Griffiths III results were supplemented by assessment with the Vineland Adaptive Behaviour Scales, on the daily living skills domain, for which his functioning was also at an average level for his age. Further analysis made it clear that there was another reason for his low scores on this scale.

The analysis pinpointed the social-emotional area where Divoc showed particular difficulty with items requiring expressive language. In the perspective-taking tasks, while he could easily pass a task where the perspective was visual (D4.1 double-sided cards), he found it really difficult to work out what another person might need to say in the theory of mind tests (D5.3 and D6.3). He could not answer questions about his personal traits or characteristics (D6.6), nor did he understand any subtleties of meaning in scenarios (D6.2 dropping plates). He found this type of task frustrating and frequently attempted avoidance or distraction. It appeared, therefore, that his difficulties with interpersonal skills were being exacerbated by his language difficulties. Divoc's mother was convinced that his behavior with other children would improve if his language improved.

The relationship between language competence and behavior problems is well established in the research literature. Children with language disorders display greater rates of problem behaviors compared with their typically developing peers, and this difference is more pronounced in older children (Curtis et al., 2018). Those with semantic and comprehension difficulties are most at risk for emotional-behavioral disorders (Helland & Helland, 2017), and those with pragmatic language difficulties are more at risk for exclusion from school (Owen, 2014). The relationship between language levels and the development of literacy skills is also well known (Pentimonti et al., 2016), and this was an area that needed to be monitored closely for Divoc.

Check Your Progress

- Why did Divoc need formulation of a program?
- What were his main areas of strength?
- What were his main areas of need?
- In which socio-emotional area did Divoc have particular difficulty?

Connecting the Dots

Divoc had experienced life-changing events such as moving country and home and not having his father living with him. Both clinical and educational concerns were focussed on his language and social functioning as he had a disorder in his use and understanding of the semantic content of language. This presentation is consistent with a diagnosis of Developmental Language Disorder. In addition, Divoc had difficulty with interpersonal relationships, an overlay of mild emotional difficulties, erratic concentration, and restless behavior. Divoc's strengths were in practical problem-solving, visual memory, self-help, and motor skills.

Charting a Plan

Divoc's mother would have liked Divoc to go to the Special Language Class, which is a highly staffed facility offering individualized teaching in very small groups with extra classroom assistants, a speech and language therapist on-site, and individual educational programs (IEPs) for every child. This is offered for the first 2 years of primary school, after which the child is enrolled in a mainstream school. This class would offer all of the skills-training components required for Divoc. Both the psychologist and speech and language therapist supported this proposal.

Divoc required a support IEP, if he was to go to a mainstream school, which will include special language input, social skills training, social-emotional skills training, anger management training, and academic support. Adjustments would need to be made in his class through more structured teaching, use of visual schedules, visual stories, and teaching social skills in a more structured manner. Early writing items which are a little challenging for Divoc should be interleaved with tasks which he finds easy, such as jigsaws and other visual puzzles, in order to support self-esteem and increase motivation.

If he did not succeed (a second time) in getting a place in the Special Language Class, multidisciplinary input in mainstream school (speech and language therapy, occupational therapy, psychology) should, if not available in the school, have been obtained from his local Early Years team and health services. Divoc would benefit from the services of a special needs assistant in the classroom and playground to help him improve his on-task behavior and to learn good interpersonal play skills as well as managing transitions and routines.

Divoc should have had a consultation to look at his vestibular and sensory functioning, also hand functioning for writing, as early academic achievement is linked with graphomotor skills (Lyons, 2020). This would give him access to any relevant educational supports needed. In Ireland where Divoc now resides, an occupational therapist is the person for this assessment.

Divoc would benefit from seeing a behavioral psychologist, and the possibility of art therapy, music therapy, play therapy, or another nonlanguage therapy could be considered, as his behavior may be linked, not only to his language difficulties, but also to family circumstances. A nonverbal medium would be good for expressing his frustrations and perhaps gently exploring his relationship with his father. Divoc's mother should be linked with relevant social services to help access any supports, both financial and social, for which she may be eligible in a new country.

Check Your Progress

- What should be on Divoc's Individual Education Plan?
- Who else should be asked to help?

Conclusion

Discussing the Key Concepts of School Readiness and of Choices of Educational Provision and School Entry

School readiness is a complex concept for which there are no nationally or internationally agreed definitions. This results in interpretations which reflect the particular views and approach of individual authors, schools, institutions, and learned societies. Differences in definition result in variance in school preparation programs, with some preschool settings concentrating narrowly on early literacy and numeracy skills, and others promoting a wider approach to life skills and educational environment, some of which also include supporting families in a broader environmental and cultural context (e.g., Gupta & Lucia, 2019).

People tend to look at school readiness from the wrong end – that is, they ask the traditional question, Does the child have the necessary skills to manage the educational and social requirements of the reception class? This is usually measured by checklists at preschool level or specialized school readiness tests. However, any method of assessing school readiness which focuses only on the child places a disproportionate emphasis on the child's abilities and skills.

A more comprehensive view of school readiness asks, Is the school ready for the child? meaning do the school and surrounding community have the resources to give a particular child the supports that are required, whether there are special needs or not? "School readiness is not just a question of whether the child is ready for school, but also whether the child's family, school and community are ready to support the child in going to school" (Christensen et al., 2020).

Attempting to define school readiness in that complex group of children who are known from an early age to be functioning in a different or developmentally unusual way from their peers becomes a complicated and often impossible task. A universal concept of school readiness can be seen as irrelevant for children with atypical development. The usefulness of items in screening tests is limited to the negative approach of making lists of what the child is failing to do. That may be adequate for the normally developing but immature or understimulated child, for whom a little help in areas that are "not quite up to standard" will suffice to bridge the developmental gap and make them ready for school. For the child with special needs, however, focusing on areas of failure will result in a very negative picture being framed. That is why a good assessment of general development is so much more useful than a school readiness screening test: It outlines the strengths of the child – what the child *can* do, as well as what they can not. The program can then be built on the child's strengths as well as on improving their areas of weaknesses.

Where a country supports full integration in schools and allocates its special needs budget to the mainstream schools, then the concept of readiness becomes redundant. "It is the responsibility of schools to meet the needs of all children at all levels of readiness" (Williams & Lerner, 2019).

A paradigm shift is, hopefully, occurring in educational thinking: from focusing on the child's level of functioning, to focusing on preparing the educational system to make individualized personal plans and curriculum adjustments suited to the child with extra needs, as well as providing blended and integrated learning opportunities for all children, both in school and in the community.

Where a country has some special services, which are apart from the regular school system, as in the case of the Special Language Class for which Divoc had applied, then a choice has to be made as to whether special services or integrated education would be better for that child. This choice will be made by parents. Informed consent will be reached after discussion with professionals who have assessed their child. Divoc's mother wished to apply for the Special Language Class for the second time, and she was supported in this by the psychologist and speech and language therapist.

In general, going to school at the same age as the other children in the reception class would appear to be the optimum placement for children. If delaying a child's entry to school is being considered, the first thing to be ascertained is whether any special programs or supports suited to the child's needs are more likely to be implemented at preschool level or at school. Keeping a child in a preschool with meagre stimulation may be a poorer option than letting them move to a school with better support, even if they seem immature for the move. On the other hand, moving a child on from a good preschool where staff are prepared to follow a program of development in the child's special areas of need, to a school with poor supports, may not be in the child's best interests. For Divoc, the positive side of an extra year in preschool was that it offered an environment where he was known and understood. However, his preschool program, while varied, did not address his particular needs in learning anger management and improving interpersonal skills. The speech therapist gave a program to his preschool to assist with language development, which was carried out as much as possible within the group. When it became known that he was not going to be offered a place in the Special Language Class, it appeared that there were no efforts made to see if his local school could make special accommodations to integrate Divoc into the reception class with supports, so he was retained in preschool. It is to be hoped that new awareness and developments in educational practice will make this less likely to happen in future.

It may be more useful to think that preparing a child for school can be described as a journey, which starts before birth with good antenatal care, and which is influenced by every inborn, environmental, and family circumstance which occurs for that child. The time of entry into school should be seen as part of a transitional continuum with the well-being of the child as its primary objective.

Check Your Progress

- Why should school readiness assessments avoid being lists of tasks the child cannot do?
- How many factors in Divoc's environment had to be taken into consideration?

Discussion Questions

- How did the move from the Czech Republic to Ireland affect Divoc? (Consider language development, house move, social and family changes, and delayed access to Early Intervention assessment.)

- Do you think that Divoc should have been sent to primary school aged 5 years 4 months, when he failed to secure a place in the Special Language Class? (Consider his age, his behavior, his language levels, the support available at preschool, and the supports potentially available to him at mainstream primary school.)
- Is the concept of school readiness a valid one for any child? (Consider the uniqueness of, and variations in, developmental maturation for each child.)

References

American Psychiatric Association. (2013). *Diagnostic and statistical manual of mental disorders* (5th ed.). https://doi.org/10.1176/appi.books.9780890425596

Christensen, D., Taylor, C. L., Hancock, K. J., & Zubrick, S. R. (2020). *School readiness is more than the child: A latent class analysis of child, family, school and community aspects of school readiness.* https://research-repository.uwa.edu.au/en/publications

Curtis, P. R., Frey, J. R., Watson, C. D., Hampton, L. H., & Roberts M. Y. (2018). Language disorders and problem behaviours: A meta-analysis. *Pediatrics, 142*(2), 1–14. https://doi.org/10.1542/peds.2017-3551

Gupta, A. & Lucia, B. (2019). School readiness in the context of inner-city Head Start centers. *Early Child Development and Care, 189*(7, 1086–1099. https://doi.org/10.1080/03004430.2017.1367925

Helland, W. A., & Helland, T. (2017). Emotional and behavioral needs in children with specific language impairment and in children with autistic spectrum disorder. *Research in Developmental Disabilities, 70,* 33–39. https://doi.org/10.1016/j.ridd.2017.08.009

Lyons, T. (2020). *Areas of the brain involved in reading and writing.* Psychology Info. https://psychology-info.com

Owen, M. (2014). *The relationship between pragmatic language competence and school exclusion: An interactionist perspective* [Unpublished doctoral dissertation]. University of Birmingham.

Pentimonti, J. M., Murphy, K., Justice, L. M., Logan, J. A., & Kaderavek, J. N. (2016). School readiness of children with language impairment: Predicting literacy skills from pre-literacy and social-behavioral dimensions. *International Journal of Language and Communication Disorders, 51*(2), 148–161. https://doi.org/10.1111/1460-6984.12193

Williams, P. G., & Lerner, M. A. (2019, August). School readiness. Council on Early Childhood and Council on School Health. *Pediatrics, 144*(2) e20191766. https://doi.org/10.1542/peds.2019-1766

World Health Organization. (2016). *International statistical classification of diseases and related health problems* (10th ed.). https://icd.who.int/browse10/2016/en

World Health Organization. (2019). *International statistical classification of diseases and related health problems* (11th ed.). https://icd.who.int/

Chapter 5

Mary: Nonstandardized Use of Griffiths III as a Qualitative Assessment of a Child Over 6 Years

Sue Bloomfield

The Context

Our pediatric team, working in the UK, was asked to assess the development of a child prior to transition from a specialist unit to a mainstream school. Mary was a girl of 6 years 5 months (77 months) with a severe physical disability secondary to *osteogenesis imperfecta* (OI). Due to her condition and frequent hospital visits, she had spent very little time in the specialist unit, but it appeared she was an able child in many areas. To start transition, it was felt it would be useful to have an overall assessment of her strengths and weaknesses to highlight which areas would require support and whether she could access a mainstream curriculum in a mainstream setting. A Griffiths III assessment was thought to be appropriate, as it is developmental in nature and assesses domains including activities of daily living as well as skills important for learning. Although she had been involved with a specialist medical team including physiotherapy, this information was not available to the assessor at this time.

Griffiths III can be used for qualitative assessment, even when children are outside the normative boundaries of the test – that is, older than the upper age limit of the test (> 6 years) or where their scores fall below the floor of the test (development quotient [DQ] < 50), by use of quartile charts.

Check Your Progress

- Why was a developmental assessment carried out?
- Why was Griffiths III used?

The Child

Mary had a severe form (type III) of OI, with recurrent fractures from an early age, bone pain, muscle weakness, and joint laxity, which had all significantly impacted on her physical development, activity level, and some abilities. Her early history was characterized by poor feeding, failure to thrive, recurrent respiratory infections, and frequent hospital visits for recurrent fractures and surgical procedures. More recently her general health was much improved, and she now had no problems with eating, drinking, or swallowing. Her sleep pattern was good. Her hearing tests were normal, and she wore spectacles for mild myopia.

Her early development had shown very slow gross motor development due partly to her muscle weakness and partly to the protective handling and environment essential to keep her safe and prevent recurrent fractures. She was nonambulant and used a wheelchair for mobility. Her fine motor development had also been slow, partly due to physical limitations with joint laxity and shortened forearms, but also reduced opportunity for typical exploration in play. Her other development in language and communication, social interaction, and problem solving appeared to follow a more typical pattern but had not been formally assessed due to her condition and frequent absences from the specialist unit.

There was no medical family history of note. She is the second of two children, and both parents were working in a professional capacity. The family had lived in the same house in the local area since Mary was born, with good family supports and no social issues.

Check Your Progress

- What are Mary's particular disabilities?

The Condition

Forlino and colleagues (2011) describe OI, often known as brittle bone disease, as a rare bone disorder characterized by bone fragility (fracturing with little-to-no trauma), short stature, long-bone deformities, bone pain, low muscle mass and weakness, persistently blue sclera (in some), and hypermobility. The prevalence of OI is estimated to be between 1 in 10,000 and 1 in 20,000 births. Shaker and colleagues (2015) have described OI as a collagen disorder with most causative genetic mutations disrupting collagen biosynthesis. It can be inherited (autosomal dominant/autosomal recessive) or occur spontaneously (de novo/mosaic mutation) and is a condition with wide variability in phenotypic expression.

Classification of OI is very complex, as described by Van Dijk and Sillence (2014) and is grouped into four or five distinct clinical phenotypes, with at least 17 different genetic mutations:

- Type I (mild),
- Type II (lethal perinatally or in first months of life),
- Type III (severe with progressive deformity with multiple fractures and wheelchair dependent),
- Type IV (moderately severe), and more recently
- Type V (similar to types I and IV).

These are the four or five phenotypes most often described in the literature, and these are attributed mainly to abnormalities of the pro-alpha-1 and pro-alpha-2 polypeptide chains of type one collagen. Some classifications try to subdivide OI into many more phenotypical groups. Mary had type III OI and was significantly affected.

Check Your Progress

- What is Mary's medical condition?
- Does it have a distinct clinical phenotype?

The Consultation

At this assessment, she was recovering from recent surgery to insert intramedullary stabilizing rods in both legs to improve her lower limb function and ability to stand, thus aiding transition from wheelchair to chair. Assessment took place with her mother. Mary was seated in a specialist, supportive, padded wheelchair with an attached tray table which was quite small and restricted the space for administering some items of the Griffiths III test (e.g., formboards). In addition, because of multiple fractures, she had quite short arms, making it difficult to reach objects when manipulation was required. Due to these constraints, some item accommodation was needed to allow some of the items to be administered. These will be discussed later.

General Observations Across the Five Subscales

Mary was very enthusiastic and engaged well with all activities even when challenging (mainly fine motor tasks). She showed good attention and listening skills plus great persistence, despite it being a long assessment on a hot day. She was sociable and chatty with a good sense of humor throughout. Figures 5.1–5.4 show the distribution of items achieved, achieved with accommodation, and not achieved, for Subscales A–D.

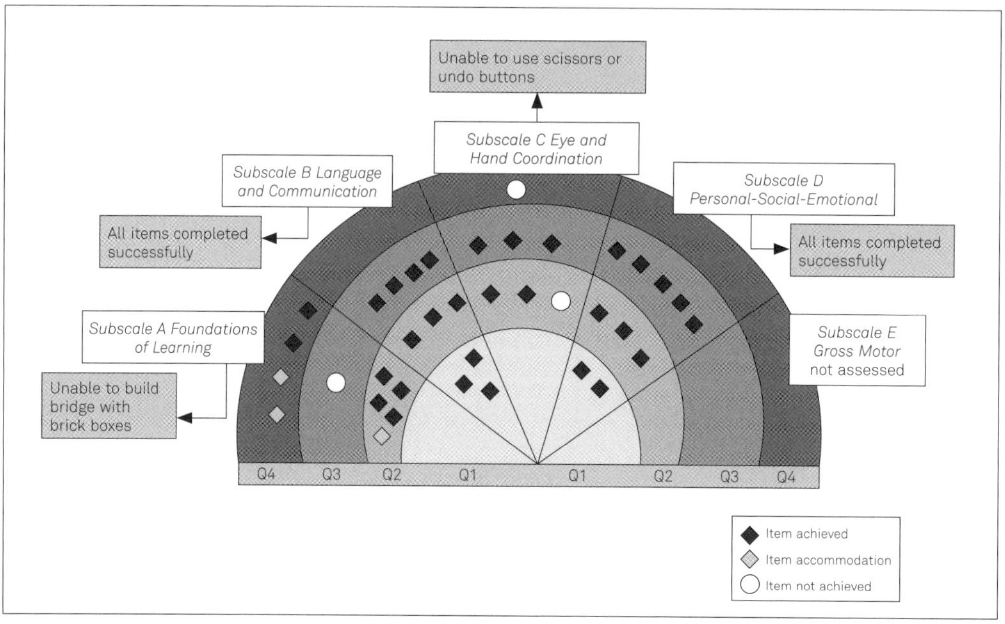

Figure 5.1. The distribution of items achieved, achieved with accommodation, and not achieved, for Subscales A–D in Year 3. Q1 = Quartile level 1, achieved by 76–100% of typically developed children by year age; Q2 = Quartile level 2, achieved by 51–75% of typically developed children by year age; Q3 = Quartile level 3, achieved by 26–50% of typically developed children by year age; Q4 = Quartile level 4, achieved by 1–25% of typically developed children by year age

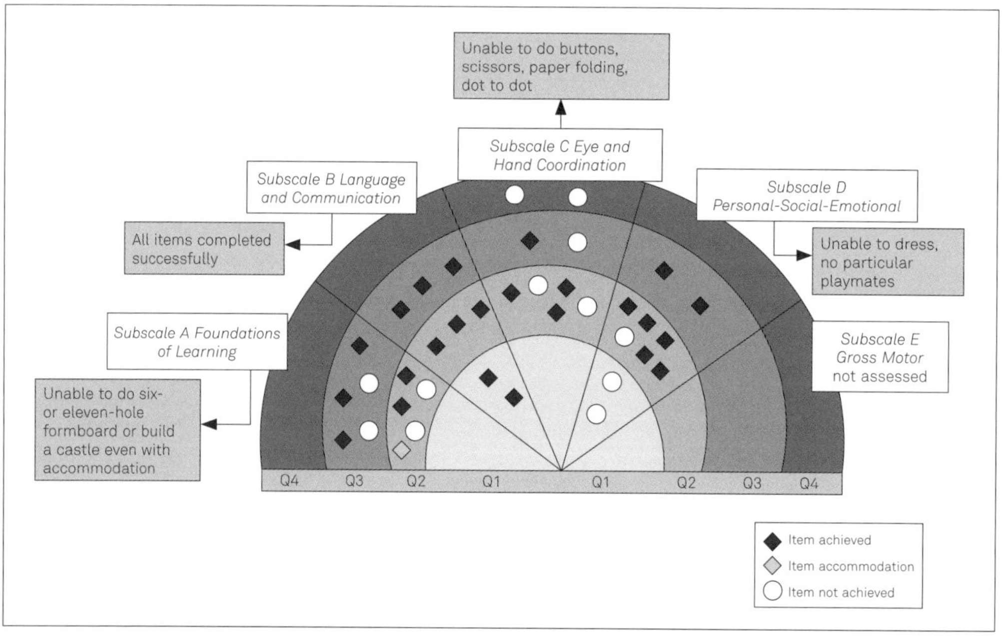

Figure 5.2. The distribution of items achieved, achieved with accommodation, and not achieved, for Subscales A–D in Year 4. Q1 = Quartile level 1, achieved by 76–100% of typically developed children by year age; Q2 = Quartile level 2, achieved by 51–75% of typically developed children by year age; Q3 = Quartile level 3, achieved by 26–50% of typically developed children by year age; Q4 = Quartile level 4, achieved by 1–25% of typically developed children by year age

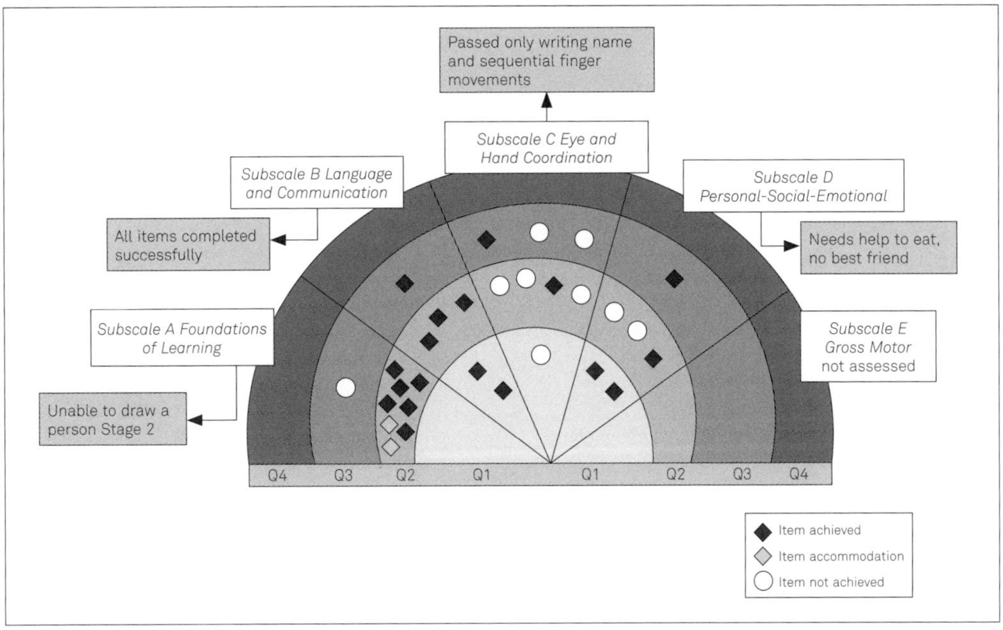

Figure 5.3. The distribution of items achieved, achieved with accommodation, and not achieved, for Subscales A–D in Year 5. Q1 = Quartile level 1, achieved by 76–100% of typically developed children by year age; Q2 = Quartile level 2, achieved by 51–75% of typically developed children by year age; Q3 = Quartile level 3, achieved by 26–50% of typically developed children by year age; Q4 = Quartile level 4, achieved by 1–25% of typically developed children by year age

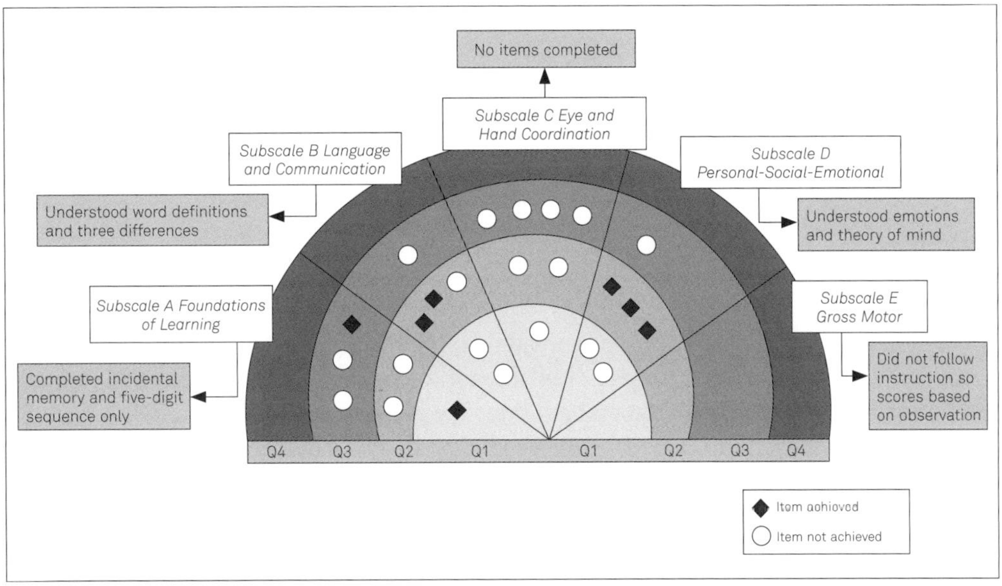

Figure 5.4. The distribution of items achieved, achieved with accommodation, and not achieved, for Subscales A–D in Year 6. Q1 = Quartile level 1, achieved by 76–100% of typically developed children by year age; Q2 = Quartile level 2, achieved by 51–75% of typically developed children by year age; Q3 = Quartile level 3, achieved by 26–50% of typically developed children by year age; Q4 = Quartile level 4, achieved by 1–25% of typically developed children by year age

Subscale A

Mary completed many of the items in this subscale (foundations of learning) including all of the quiet book items. She had little difficulty with numeracy and digit sequences, spot-the-difference, left/right discrimination, patternmaking, and the first picture arrangement. She was able to hold the dabber, and although she marked the page lightly, it was sufficient for successful completion of the two object hunt items.

For tasks where there is not a significant fine motor element, she passed items in the third quartile of Year 6, skills achieved at an approximate age of 66–69 months. Her performance, however, was very patchy due to her problems with fine motor skills as seen with the brick box and formboard items. She had problems with these tasks involving fine motor constructs where she had difficulty in Year 3 where children of approximate age 31–33 months would be competent.

Interestingly, she managed the patternmaking sequence where motor planning and visual concept constructs are more important than fine motor manipulation.

In summary, she had achieved levels of skill for memory, ways of thinking, and problem solving, in the range expected for children in Year 6, whereas other skills with a fine motor component were more immature, at a Year 2–3 level.

Subscale B

Language and communication was an area of real strength for Mary. She was chatty, and showed a good amount of reciprocal conversation. She listened and attended well to the questions. She completed all of the items to the end of Year 5. She understood all three differences and word definitions for Year 6 but had more difficulty with creating a narrative or using three or more descriptive sentences for the large picture. Her language skills for both receptive and expressive language were in the second quartile of Year 6, skills achieved at an approximate age of 64–66 months.

Subscale C

Eye and hand coordination was the area which posed the most difficulty for her. She was able build a tower of eight bricks and threaded all 11 beads successfully. She showed persistence with this task even though it was difficult for her and took some time. There was no tremor, and she had a good fine pincer grip. She put the pegs in the cup individually in under 20 seconds but not the pegs in the peg board in under 60 seconds (speed of movement). She managed the playdough sausage and ball but neither paper folding item. She drew a horizontal stroke, a circle and cross Stage 1, but not the more mature shapes. She wrote her name using the chunky pencil in an immature tripod grip with minimal pencil pressure, but the result was legible. She preferred to use the dabber for draw a person. She did not pass the dot-to-dot or trail items as she had poor pencil control.

Complex motor tasks such as construction pieces and lacing were not completed. She was unable to handle scissors or undo any buttons even the single large button. Her fine motor skills were generally at Year 4 level, skills achieved at an approximate age of 40–45 months, but quite patchy. She had difficulties, however, at a much earlier stage not being able to achieve any scissors or button items. Graphomotor tasks were a challenge.

Subscale D

Personal-social-emotional constructs were an area of strength for Mary in many areas, as she had a good understanding of feelings and emotions for both herself and others. Activities of daily living were still a big challenge for her, including dressing, undressing, and eating without assistance. She had good bladder and bowel control both day and night but needed a considerable amount of help with using the bathroom. She was unable to identify a best friend or even one or two playmates; this is not unexpected with her lack of nursery and school experience and frequent periods in hospital. Her social and emotional understanding were in the second quartile of Year 6 skills achieved at an approximate age 64–66 months. Her daily living skills were at a more immature level, in the first quartile of Year 4; an approximate age of 37–39 months, due to her fine motor difficulties.

Subscale E

Due to her condition and recent surgery, gross motor skills were not assessed.

Accommodations Required to Complete Some Test Items

As described at the beginning of the assessment, and due to Mary's physical limitations, some test items were administered in a nonstandard way and not exactly according to the Griffiths III Administration Manual instructions, to allow her to complete a task. This particularly related to enabling her to reach objects (see Box 5.1).

Box 5.1. Accommodations required to complete some test items

- Stacking pieces for the six- and eleven-hole formboards at each side instead at the upper edge of the formboard to enable her to reach them
- Ensuring all items using the quiet book are within easy reach for example reassembling the train puzzle
- Helping her physically to put buttons on the memory house in the places as directed by her
- Folding pages and moving them sequentially for both object hunt tasks so she could reach them with the dabber to successfully complete the item
- Using the dabber rather than the chunky pencil for some drawing items as it is easier to hold and requires less pressure to make a mark
- Ensuring objects for following instructions in the language subscale (particularly one-, two-, and three-part commands) are easy to reach so this does not distract from the instruction

Check Your Progress

- Why is it important to consider the constraints to the assessment?
- Are all of Mary's skills at the same developmental level?
- Why are accommodations used?

Connecting the Dots

Griffiths III could not be used in a standardized way as Mary was older than 6 years, and some accommodation of items administrated was required. Therefore, standardized scores and base rate significance between subscales could not be used to describe her performance. Very good qualitative information, however, was obtained and has been summarized in Table 5.1 and illustrated visually in Figures 5.1 to 5.4. These contributed to forward planning.

Table 5.1. Age equivalence using quartile charts

Subscale A	67–69 months for tasks with constructs of ways of thinking, memory, and skills for learning 31–33 months for tasks having additional constructs of motor planning and fine motor skills
Subscale B	64–66 months for tasks with constructs of receptive and expressive language, verbal reasoning, and semantic development
Subscale C	40–45 months for tasks with constructs of fine motor and bilateral coordination, speed, and graphomotor
Subscale D	64–66 months for tasks with constructs of social and emotional understanding 37–39 months for daily living skills

Mary had many strengths which would enable her to have success in a mainstream setting. She was enthusiastic and showed reasonably good attention and listening skills, plus persistence and determination even with challenging tasks. She had no difficulty with auditory or visual memory, numeracy skills, or problem solving where there was not a fine motor construct involved. She had reasonable visual discrimination for visual materials such as the large picture and spot-the-difference.

She had good skills in both receptive and expressive language. She was keen to communicate and was socially engaging with an appropriate degree of social understanding. These were all skills which were needed for her to make the transition to mainstream schooling and to access the curriculum.

She did, however, have difficulties with a range of motor tasks, particularly where there were fine motor or graphomotor elements involved. These were delayed compared with her verbal and cognitive skills. She had joint laxity and muscle weakness which made it hard for her to put sufficient pressure on paper. Pencil control was poor. Activities of daily living needed significant support. She was nonambulant and wheelchair dependent.

She had a complex medical condition which made her physically very vulnerable. OI is a complex disorder which is best managed by a multidisciplinary team – if possible, from a specialist center (Marr et al., 2017). There are a number of these in the UK, and they also provide outreach services. The team includes a pediatrician, often the first involved for diagnosis and management of conditions including respiratory or gastrointestinal problems and pain management. An orthopedic surgeon is important for fracture management, both for acute fractures and prophylactic intervention to prevent deformity. A neurosurgeon may be needed for issues including hydrocephalus and potential spinal cord damage.

Physiotherapy and occupational therapy input are vital in the early baby and toddler years, as well as later. Other professionals on the team include a clinical nurse specialist, speech and language therapist, dietitian, psychologist, and social worker. With the consent of parents or carers, liaison with the school from the medical team is important to give necessary information and training.

Good information is available through the Brittle Bone Society, who provide support and trusted advice and information. Patients, families, and carers are encouraged to use these resources. The Pediatric Osteogenesis Imperfecta National Team (POINT) was formed with an aim to provide a forum for clinicians in the UK with an interest in OI to meet and share information. Living in the UK, Mary luckily had access to these services. Areas needing support for transition included:

- Forward planning with school to ensure classroom and facilities are wheelchair accessible,
- Safe environment while allowing for graded exercise and activity and suitable space for this,
- Trained support staff in school for daily living tasks, exercise programs, and classroom activities when needed,
- Appropriate seating at desk,
- Aids for graphomotor skills and accessing the curriculum, and
- Peer group integration.

Charting a Plan

Further assessment of Mary and the school setting by a physiotherapist was vital. An excellent consensus paper by Mueller and colleagues (2018) describes the input needed. They use the *International Classification of Functioning, Disability and Health of Children and Youth* (ICF-CY; WHO, 2007) as a framework to make recommendations in 17 areas for input. It is essential to ensure the physical environment is safe to reduce the risk of further fractures while encouraging activity. Physiotherapy needs to consider energy conservation, positioning, joint protection, and environmental access. The goals are to improve strength, stamina, and mobility; to progress to independent self-care skills; and to allow children to have fun being active as far as possible. Mary might have required regular positioning and exercise during the school day.

Mary was wheelchair dependent for mobility at that time, and therefore access to all areas of the school needed to be appropriate, particularly classroom and toilets, with building adaptation if necessary. Appropriate supportive seating would have been essential for her to access tabletop materials in the classroom. Further detailed assessment by an occupational therapist would ascertain the type of program and adaptations to help her access the curriculum. She would require assistance with daily living skills such as dressing and undressing, but particularly with toileting and at mealtimes. She might also require significant support to compensate for her graphomotor and other fine motor difficulties, to allow her to access the curriculum at a level commensurate with her other abilities. The type of aids needed would have depended on the detailed occupational therapy assessment, but they would normally range from simple items such as pencil grips and Lycra gloves to improve pencil control, to a range of assisted technologies including tablet computer, other computers, and keyboards, which might be needed in the future. Useful guides for educators for children with physical difficulties have been produced which outline many helpful options (Torreno, 2011).

Mary would also have benefited from a program, for school and home, to encourage graphomotor skills and achieve independent daily living skills. Another area to consider would have been the impact of OI on everyday life; her friendships were not yet fully established. She was adept socially with adults, but her lack of opportunity for peer group interaction needed to be considered when helping her integrate. Psychological support is also needed by some children (Marr et al., 2017).

Check Your Progress

- Why is input from a physiotherapist very important for Mary?
- What adaptations will be needed in school?
- Who should provide guidance to the school?

Conclusion

The above case study shows that Griffiths III, a comprehensive child-friendly developmental assessment which covers five avenues of learning, can be used as a qualitative assessment to give a profile of a child's strengths and weaknesses even when it is used outside the normal boundaries of the test. The subscales can be used independently to look at specific aspects of development.

Developmental tests are mostly standardized on typically developing children and do not take into consideration the impact of physical or other difficulties on successful test completion. A child may conceptually understand a task and would be able to pass a test item if unhindered by physical or other problems.

A number of tests have been designed for assessing children with specific conditions (see the section Resources). The ICF-CY (WHO, 2007) focuses on aspects of functional skill level and is useful for planning therapeutic intervention, caregiver assistance, and adaptive equipment. There are many batteries of occupational therapy and physiotherapy assessments used by therapists which can all contribute to intervention plans.

Griffiths III in one assessment gives a holistic overview of a child's development and can be used in a nonstandard way (in this case for a child older than 6 years and with a physical disability) where numerical scores cannot be obtained, by use of the quartile charts. Item accommodation is sometimes needed to enable successful completion of some test items, but an approximate measure of where a child's skills are can be obtained and gives a profile of strengths and weaknesses. This widens the applicability of Griffiths III beyond the normative boundaries of the test. In addition, the assessment is used to obtain valuable observational information about a child (including attention, listening skills, perseverance, enthusiasm, and imagination), which all add to the picture. Recommendations to help support the child can then be made using such qualitative information where numerical information is not available.

Discussion Questions

- How much item accommodation should be used to enable a child to complete a test?
- Could test items be adapted to tablet computer format to enable a child with physical difficulties to more easily pass test items?
- If so, which items?
- For Mary, how successful do you think integration into mainstream schooling will be?
- What are the barriers to her success?

Resources

Self-Help Organizations

The Brittle Bone Society offers support and advice to parents of children with all types of OI. Website: https://www.brittlebone.org/.

Tests Assessing Specific Areas of Development

Raven, J. C., Raven, J., & Court, L. (2019). *Raven's Colour Progressive Matrices (CPM) for use with children and elderly people*. Pearson.
These are designed now for children aged 4 to 11 years of age, older persons, and mentally and physically impaired individuals. This test contains colored and black-and-white matrices with the individual finding the missing piece from a selection. They are independent of language and reading and writing skills. They assume normal vision and visual processing and look at deductive and nonverbal problem solving.

Reynell, J. (1979). *Manual for the Reynell-Zinkin scales, developmental scales for young visually handicapped children: Part 1. mental development*. NFER – Nelson.
These were devised for specific areas of difficulty and rate of individual progress and are designed to help create an early intervention plan for children with visual impairment, age range: birth to 4 years.

Tellegen, P., & Laros, J. (2014). *The SON-R 2-8 (Snijders-Ooman Non-Verbal Intelligence Test)*. Hogrefe. This test is applied without the use of verbal or written instruction for the assessment of children with hearing impairment, learning difficulties, or language and communication barriers. Age range: 2–8 years.

References

Forlino, A., Cabral, W., Barnes, A., & Marini, J. (2011). New perspectives on osteogenesis imperfecta. *Nature Reviews Endocrinology, 7*(9), 540–557. https://doi.org/10.1038/nrendo.2011.81

Marr, C., Seasman, A., & Bishop, N. (2017). Managing the patient with osteogenesis imperfecta: A multidisciplinary approach. *Journal of Multidisciplinary Healthcare, 10,* 145–155. https://doi.org/10.2147/JMDH.S113483

Mueller, B., Engelbert, R., Baratta-Ziska, F., Bartels, B., Blanc, N., Brizola, E., Fraschini, P., Hill, C., Marr, C., Mills, L., Montpetit, K., Pacey, V., Rodriquez- Molina, M., Schuuring, M., Verhille, C., de Vries, O., Kwong Yeung, E., & Semler, O. (2018). Consensus statement on physical rehabilitation in children and adolescents with osteogenesis imperfecta. *Orphanet Journal of Rare Diseases, 13*(158). https://doi.org/10.1186/s13023-018-0905-4

Shaker, J., Albert, C., Fritz, J., & Harris, G. (2015). Recent developments in osteogenesis imperfecta. *F1000Research, 4*(F1000 Faculty Rev), 681. https://doi.org/10.12688/f1000research.6398.1

Torreno, S. (2011). A guide to inclusion & teaching strategies for students with physical disabilities. *Bright Hub Education, 2020*(946). https://www.brighthubeducation.com

Van Dijk, F., & Sillence, D. (2014). Osteogenesis imperfecta: Clinical diagnosis, nomenclature and severity assessment. *American Journal of Medical Genetics, 164*(6), 1470–1481. https://doi.org/10.1002/ajmg.a.36545

World Health Organization. (2007). *International classification of functioning, disability and health for children and youth (ICF-CY).*

Chapter 6

Poppy: A Child With Hearing Impairment and Congenital Cytomegalovirus Infection

Jennifer Jansen

The Context

I am a clinical psychologist working in a university clinic based in South Africa. This case study describes a girl called Poppy who had a hearing impairment, possibly due to congenital *cytomegalovirus* (CMV) infection. Poppy's relatively late diagnosis of bilateral hearing loss was reported by health care professionals to play a significant role in her present general developmental delay. Of greatest concern to the health care professionals was her slow pace of both receptive and expressive language acquisition. Other possible reasons reported included both environmental and cognitive impingements.

Poppy was a 3-year-5-month-old English-speaking girl residing in an impoverished environment in South Africa. She had been diagnosed with a moderate bilateral hearing loss at the age of 2 years 10 months, and the only intervention prior to her developmental assessment was fitting her with hearing aids and irregular speech therapy sessions due to lack of parental cooperation. Another disabling factor was that Poppy's hearing aids were frequently in need of repair, resulting in no amplification of sound for lengthy periods of time.

She was referred by her speech therapist for a developmental assessment as Poppy displayed limited linguistic progress despite intermittent therapeutic interventions. She needed further evaluation for appropriate educational intervention. The objective of the assessment carried out by the clinical psychologist was to examine Poppy's current developmental functioning and provide an intervention plan for the future.

The Child

Poppy was born preterm by emergency cesarean section at 33 weeks of gestation. She weighed 1,200 g (2 lb 10 oz) and was jaundiced. Maternal preeclampsia and intrauterine growth restriction were recorded in her file. Poppy was noted to be hypotonic and anemic at birth. Her developmental milestones were not clearly remembered by her parents, but comments made by them indicated a general developmental delay.

Poppy was an only child and had not attended any type of formalized learning environment as her parents did not see this as a priority. The language spoken at home was English, but the larger community where Poppy spent most of her time, spoke a mixture of three languages – English, Afrikaans, and isiXhosa. The young parents never completed their schooling, and the family lived on a menial income from the two parental incomes,

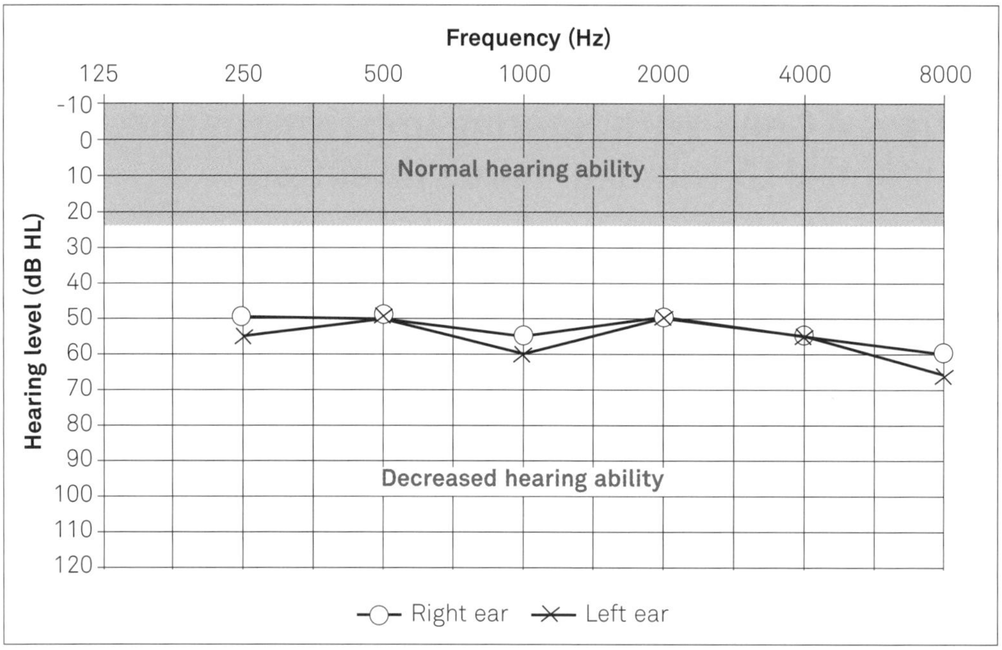

Figure 6.1. Poppy's audiogram attached to her referral, indicating moderate sensorineural loss in both ears. Vertical axis represents the volume measured in decibels (dB) while the horizontal axis represents sound frequency measured in Hertz (Hz)

while an aunt cared for Poppy during the week. The parents reported inconsistent discipline at home, as they were tired after work. Two months before her developmental evaluation, an ear, nose, and throat specialist had confirmed hearing loss and bone malformations in both ears, as well as evidence of past CMV infection in both the mother and Poppy.

Poppy's audiogram was attached to the referral and indicated a moderate sensorineural loss in both ears. The results are represented on Figure 6.1 where the vertical axis represents the volume measured in decibels (dB) while the horizontal axis represents sound frequency measured in Hertz (Hz). The results are globally recorded on the audiogram by means of "O"s for the right ear and "X"s for the left one.

The audiogram was helpful as frequencies between 300 and 500 Hz are most commonly used in conversation, and her deficit fell within this range. Based on the results of the audiogram, Poppy had been fitted with hearing aids. Generally speaking, the more markings below 25 dB, which are frequencies normally used in conversation, the more difficult it is to hear what is being said. Poppy should have been able to hear low-frequency words if there is no background noise but would need amplification of sound to grasp speech. However, she was exposed to three different languages on a daily basis and not able to grasp the need for language. This may be indicative of comorbid cognitive impairment.

Check Your Progress

- Is Poppy's hearing loss likely to affect her language development?

The Condition

The typical clinical symptoms of symptomatic congenital CMV are found in 10–20% of infected neonates and include intrauterine growth restriction, microcephaly, hepatosplenomegaly, petechiae, jaundice, chorioretinitis, thrombocytopenia, anemia, and/or other atypical findings (Ornoy & Diav-Citrin, 2006). CMV usually results in different neurodevelopmental sequelae such as mental retardation, motor impairment, sensorineural hearing loss, or visual impairment, which may occur even in infants who are free of symptoms at birth (Ornoy & Diav-Citrin, 2006). Most infants born with severe neonatal symptoms of congenital CMV are born to mothers with primary infection in pregnancy (Ornoy & Diav-Citrin, 2006.)

Congenital CMV infection may result from transplacental acquisition of either a primary or recurrent maternal infection (Centers for Disease Control and Prevention, 2020). Preterm infants who lack antibodies to CMV may become infected perinatally by exposure to infected secretions. As in most countries, screening is not carried out in South Africa (Lazzarotto et al., 2020). CMV remains a leading cause of congenital infections worldwide (Gunkel et al., 2018).

Check Your Progress

- What developmental sequelae are seen after congenital CMV?

The Consultation

Griffiths III was used to assess Poppy's current developmental functioning and took place over two sessions because she became fatigued during testing. She struggled to understand what was expected of her and would then abandon the task. Her hearing aids distracted her when they whistled, and she would then stop the task and focus on trying stop the sound by placing her hands over the earmolds.

It was difficult to determine whether Poppy could understand the instructions or if she was unable to execute the items presented. For this reason, the instructions had to be repeated several times without excessive nonverbal demonstrations which would have invalidated the test.

Assessment Results Across the Five Subscales

Considering the results on Griffiths III holistically, Poppy's scores fell within the extremely low range, with a developmental age equivalent of 25 months. The scores obtained depicted that Poppy was functioning 16 months below her chronological age at that time. Her overall score indicated a development quotient of 50, which placed her below the first percentile and implied that her general development could be described as poorer than 99% of children aged 41 months (3 years 5 months). From Poppy's low scores across the five subscales, it could reasonably be assumed that there were significant developmental delays across all domains assessed. The scores supported concerns about future development and school placement. Table 6.1 shows the raw score conversions.

Table 6.1. Conversion of raw scores to scaled scores

Subscale	Scaled score	Development quotient	Percentile	Age equivalent
Subscale A	4	66	2	26 months
Subscale B	0	< 50	< 1	< 21 months
Subscale C	6	77	7	31 months
Subscale D	3	62	1	26 months
Subscale E	6	77	2	32 months
General development	0	50	< 1	25 months

To analyze the patterns regarding Poppy's skill deficits on all subscales, the items achieved or not achieved were analyzed on the Griffiths III Quartile Charts to evaluate her relative strengths and weaknesses. Poppy's functioning on the Year 3 is represented in Figure 6.2.

Base rates offer extra information on the difference in scaled score between subscales. Significant differences were found between Subscales A and B, Subscales B and C, and Subscales B and E. Qualitative analysis of the results indicated that Poppy's limited language acquisition and possible cognitive and environmental factors seemed to have influenced her scores across all developmental domains.

Constructs that were problematic on Subscale A were ways of thinking, play, auditory memory, and auditory processing. This was understandable as she had a hearing loss, and language is integral to the development of these constructs. Her inability to respond to questions regarding size concepts such as "big" and "small," as well as spatial concepts such as "Show me the cupcake in the 'middle,'" highlighted compromised concept formation. The constructs that evaluated play may have been influenced by limited cognitive ability and/or social isolation.

There were items that Poppy might have completed, but she did not understand the instruction given. She was unable to repeat simple digit series, which could have been the result of poor auditory processing, or problems with auditory memory or concentration, or an inability to hear. She successfully completed elementary formboards after demonstration, indicating that she had developed rudimentary visual imitation skills, which are essential skills for future learning. Throughout the assessment, tasks requiring concentration and reasoning were met with resistance.

On Subscale B, language and communication, Poppy's approach to task taking indicated that she had not developed skills for listening and did not understand the necessity for communication. She found it difficult to make her needs known verbally, leading to her parents finding it difficult to understand her, and regressed behaviors that were difficult

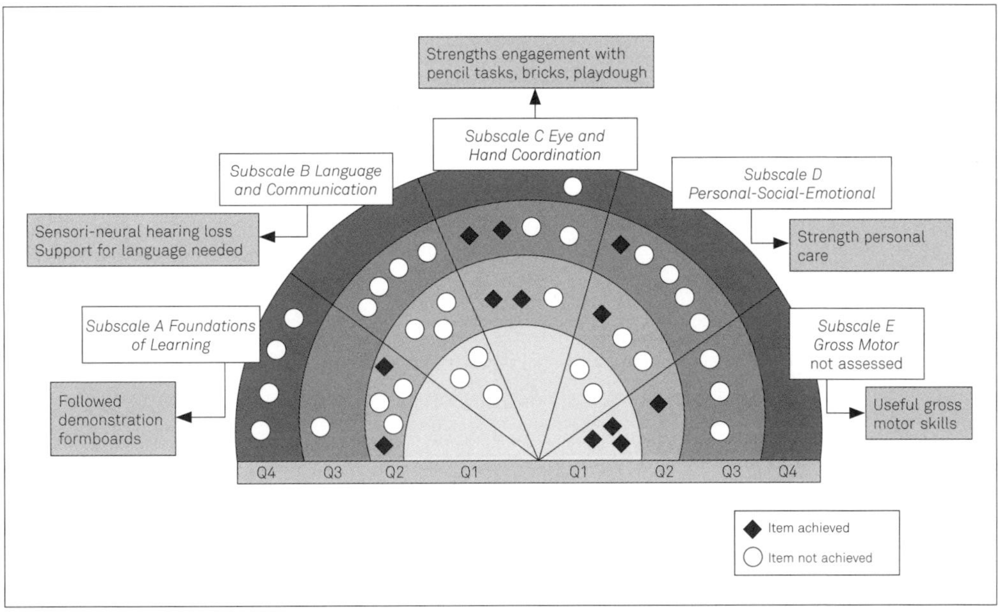

Figure 6.2. Distribution of items achieved or not achieved using the Griffiths III Quartile Chart Year 3. Q1 = Quartile level 1, achieved by 76–100% of typically developed children by year age; Q2 = Quartile level 2, achieved by 51–75% of typically developed children by year age; Q3 = Quartile level 3, achieved by 26–50% of typically developed children by year age; Q4 = Quartile level 4, achieved by 1–25% of typically developed children by year age

for the parents to handle. Her receptive language seemed better developed than her expressive skills, as she reacted to a few simple commands confined to pointing to everyday objects used in the home environment, such as cup, dog, and spoon, but not to those that were symbolically represented. She did however respond to verbs such as "jump" and "throw," but only when the actions were demonstrated.

Her limited receptive vocabulary and communicative intent, together with her permanent moderate bilateral hearing loss and impoverished environment, had played a significant role in her inability to attain basic expressive language skills. Poppy's expressive verbalizations were confined to a few single words, and no two-word utterances were expressed during the assessment. She had no desire to imitate words which are imperative for vocabulary development and expressive language.

Her Subscale C scores (for eye and hand coordination) suggested that this domain, although poorly developed, was a relative strength. She did complete one item in Year 4, as she was able to copy a circle (Stage 1). Poppy found fine motor items such as threading beads, undoing and fastening buttons difficult. Although she did engage in pencil and paper tasks, her execution of these activities did not go beyond rudimentary representations of the symbolic presentations.

On Subscale D, personal-social-emotional, Poppy responded to her name but did not give her name on request. She did not respond to the question, Are you a boy or a girl? Poppy had been toilet trained and partook in basic self-care tasks such as pulling up her elasticized pants. Her parents reported that she did not interact appropriately with peers and tended to resort to insular activities where no demands were made on her. She was an only child, with limited opportunities provided to engage with other children. Poppy did not pass items that require identification of basic emotions, expressions of thoughts and feeling, and participation in group play.

On Subscale E, gross motor, Poppy was able to perform basic gross motor and visual-spatial activities, such as throwing a short tennis ball and walking up and down stairs. Her balance posed a problem, which might be attributed to aberrant equilibrium responses and concomitant vestibular dysfunction often found in children with a bilateral sensorineural hearing loss (Masuda & Kaga, 2014). Poppy was unable to stand on one foot for 3 seconds or hop on one foot. She had midline difficulties such as crossing knees and feet when seated. Although her gross motor skills are not at an age-appropriate level, this area of functioning was a relative strength for her. Outdoor play also needs to form part of her intervention plan.

Check Your Progress

- Why were the Griffiths III Quartile Charts used?
- How did Poppy's hearing loss affect the assessment?
- Did she demonstrate difficulties which were not caused by her hearing loss?

Connecting the Dots

Poppy was a 3-year-5-month-old girl with a bilateral hearing loss, who was functioning in the far-below-average range on all of the subscales, and below the 50th quotient on the language and communication subscale. She presented with both internal and external barriers that would have the potential to impact on cognitive functioning and future learning.

Although her hearing had been amplified with state-funded bilateral aids, these devices were reported to often be broken. Scarcity of audiology appointments had meant that Poppy was still wearing the original earmolds which were ill-fitting at the time of the assessment and urgently needed to be replaced, as she was growing.

Her young parents had never completed their schooling and appeared to lack some basic understanding of child development. Thus, parenting was inconsistent and reactive. Limited exposure to goal-directed play and educational materials *had* possibly *also contributed* to Poppy's poor performance.

There had been no consistent carryover of new material learned in the individual speech therapy to the parents, and this had led to a disconnect between new information learned and practice at home. This had also led to interventions being fragmented, resulting in poor progress.

Poppy's strengths	Poppy's needs
• Engagement with pencil tasks, bricks, playdough • Personal care	• Management of her hearing impairment • Multiprofessional input for therapy and teaching

Charting a Plan

There had been limited interventions to assist Poppy's developmental progress. The constructs highlighted on the assessment as not achieved can be used to assist with future intervention. This needs to be process-based, with regular evaluations by the professionals working with her.

Application should be made to a mainstream school with separate classes for children who have partial hearing loss. Placement at a school for the deaf should not be considered immediately, as she is still young and, if placed correctly, will have an opportunity to learn language in a classroom environment. This placement may need to be reassessed in the future, as it is difficult to make this decision at this stage of her development.

A wider range of professionals should contribute to her intervention program; hence special school placement was needed in South Africa. Such a team would include the parents, specialist teachers, and professionals who have specialist training to carry out assessment of need, as well as the technical knowledge to undertake the necessary teaching approaches. These professionals need to interact with each other on a regular basis to prevent siloed interventions.

Practical Aspects

Correctly adjusted hearing aids is the core of any auditory intervention and integral to intervention with regard to hearing (Turan, 2012). Poppy's parents and aunt need to be made aware of their responsibilities in the efficient use of the hearing aids. The parents need to be assisted in hearing aid use which would help them to gain confidence in dealing with the devices. Young children are often not capable of signaling when there are problems with incoming sound. Poppy's vision also needs to be assessed.

Intervention Sessions

Initially time should be given to knowledge dissemination. Adults working with Poppy need to understand voice clashes, when one or more person is talking (Clark, 2007). They need to know that hearing aids do not restore hearing to normal levels and that background noise has a deteriorative effect on speech sounds, as well as knowing about the negative effect of hearing aid microphone distance on speech perception (Clark, 2007).

While waiting for placement in a mainstream preschool with classes for partially hearing children, Poppy needs to be involved in home-based activities with an emphasis on expanding her vocabulary and paying attention to imitation of words. These could include bathing. In this situation she would be provided with the opportunity to learn to recognize and name body parts, as well as dressing, and in so doing, learn to name the different clothing items. Such activities would provide a regular opportunity for learning both vocabulary and language. During interactions, there must be an insistence that Poppy imitate words spoken. By talking about language and vocabulary pertinent to the activity she is busy with, the parents would be most likely to provide meaningful language input to the child.

Providing her with experiential routine activities, she would be more likely to regularly associate words with objects, and in this way expand her vocabulary. The level of difficulty could be incrementally increased as her vocabulary and length of sentence usage expanded. An example would be "Give me the banana," a command requiring receptive language. The following level would be "What is this?" The expressive response will be "banana." Then a verb could be added receptively such as in the phrase "Peel the banana." The command could be further extended to "What are you doing?" Later, household activities such sorting the washing, cleaning, and bathing could provide opportunities to teach vocabulary, fine motor skills, and routine.

Sessions at this stage of her development should take the form of guiding Poppy's parents to work with her so that she realizes that listening and speaking are a way of life, and their awareness is heightened as to how much they already knew (Turan, 2012). Observing parents interacting with their child serves several purposes, and arrangements need to be made with the parents' employers to be present at some of the sessions or until she was placed in school. The sessions would also provide an opportunity to monitor the Poppy's progress; the overall aim being to lead the parents toward competence and independence. This needed to be reinstated by all who worked with her.

The other developmental skills Poppy has not developed could be built into these sessions, including activities such as threading, learning colors, and basic interactive games. While participating in all of the above activities, skill competency and language could then be simultaneously achieved. Singing, reciting rhymes, and simple repetitive songs with hand actions are to be recommended to widen her listening experience. The parents need to learn that any activity can provide opportunities for learning vocabulary and language.

A preschool environment would give Poppy the opportunity to improve her social skills. Poppy has difficulty recognizing emotions and as a result receives negative reactions from the adults in her world and suffered from social isolation. This aspect could be mediated in a formalized learning environment.

Check Your Progress

- How were the activities chosen to progress Poppy's development?
- Why was a school for the deaf not suggested at this stage?
- What are voice clashes and how can they be prevented?

Conclusion

Poppy has a bilateral sensorineural hearing loss presumably as a result of congenital CMV infection. Her assessment showed that she has significantly delayed development in all domains but particularly in language and communication, and thus provided developmental information to guide the way forward for Poppy's education. All health care professionals need to be involved at this stage of her development, as it is not yet clear if her hearing impairment is her only educational challenge.

Discussion Questions

- Who would make the decision as to whether Poppy's language development would improve should cochlear implants be considered?
- What would the criteria for a cochlear implant be based on, other than speech and language progress?
- Do you think her current cognitive ability would impede the benefits of such an operation?
- If and when would sign language be considered, and on what grounds?
- What are the advantages and disadvantages of signing and/or learning spoken language?
- What methods could be put in place to encourage better parenting of Poppy?
- To what extent was her poor language ability affecting her general developmental functioning in each of the five domains assessed on Griffiths III?

References

Centers for Disease Control and Prevention. (2020, August 18). *Cytomegalovirus (CMV) and congenital CMV infection.* https://www.cdc.gov/cmv/index.html

Clark, M. (2007). *A practical guide to quality interaction with children who have hearing loss.* Plural.

Gunkel, J., de Vries, L. S., Jongmans, M., Koopman-Esseboom, C., van Haastert, I. C., Eijsermans, M. C., van Stam, C., van Zanten, B. G., Wolfs, T. F., & Nijman, J. (2018). Outcome postnatal cytomegalovirus infection. *Pediatrics 141*(2). https://doi.org/10.1542/ped.2017-0635

Lazzarotto, T., Blázquez-Gamero, D., Delforge, L., Foulon, I., Luck, S., Modrow, S., & Leruez-Ville, M. (2020). Congenital cytomegalovirus infection: A narrative review of the issues in screening and management from a panel of European experts. *Frontier Pediatrics, 8*(13). https://doi.org/10.3389/fped.2020.00013

Masuda, T., & Kaga, K. (2014). Relationship between acquisition of motor function and vestibular function in children with bilateral severe hearing loss. *Acta Oto-Laryngologica, 134*(7), 672–678. https://doi.org/10.3109/00016489.2014.890290

Ornoy, A., & Diav-Citrin, O. (2006). Fetal effects of primary and secondary cytomegalovirus infection in pregnancy. *Reproductive Toxicology, 21*(4), 399–409. https://doi.org/10.1016/j.reprotox.2005.02.002

Turan, Z. (2012). *Early intervention with children who have a hearing loss: Role of the professional and parent participation.* IntechOpen. https://doi.org/10.5772/32769

Zone 2

Zone 2: Children With Dominant Symptoms of the Autistic Spectrum	
Chapter 7	Hugo: A Brazilian Child Diagnosed With Autism Spectrum Disorder
Chapter 8	Jamie: Assessing a Child With High Functioning Autism
Chapter 9	Eli: Assessing a Child With Low Functioning Autism
Chapter 10	Victor: Resilience in the COVID-19 Pandemic

Chapter 7

Hugo: A Brazilian Child Diagnosed With Autism Spectrum Disorder

Amanda Tragueta Ferreira-Vasques and Dionísia Aparecida Cusin Lamônica

The Context

The following case was attended to in a private clinic by the first author, a child speech-language pathology and audiology therapist, working in the area of child development in Brazil. Both authors are researchers in language development and child development. We carried out the translation, cross-cultural adaptation of the Griffiths III Development Scale, and the standardization for the 0- to 24-month age group in the Brazilian Portuguese language. We are currently conducting the standardization for the age group of 25 to 72 months.

The case study presented here is about the evaluation of a boy, Hugo, who was Brazilian and 23 months old. The family sought a neuropediatrician, as the child was still not speaking. After clinical evaluation, the neuropediatrician gave a diagnosis of *autism spectrum disorder* (ASD). As part of the medical management, the physician referred the child for speech therapy evaluation.

Objectives of the Case

The objectives with this child were

- To understand the history of Hugo's development,
- To read about ASD and to know more about the child who was being evaluated, regarding his potentials and limitations,
- To associate subjective and objective clinical assessments, using standardized and normalized assessment instruments for child development, such as Griffiths III, and
- To understand the diagnostic reasoning that should be used to develop the intervention plan.

The Child

At the first meeting, the family reported their reason for seeking speech therapy evaluation (absence of speech), and data were collected on the child's history and the family's socioeconomic status, such as education, and socioeconomic level.

Parents had completed high school, and they confirmed their medium-low socioeconomic status. During the planned pregnancy, Hugo's mother had had hypothyroidism and gestational diabetes, controlled with medication and diet. She had also had a urinary tract infection treated with antibiotics. Hugo was the son of nonconsanguineous parents. The delivery was full-term and normal. His weight and height at birth were 3,060 g (6 lbs 12 oz) and 49.5 cm (19.5 in.), respectively, with Apgar scores 8/9. He had neonatal icterus and was hospitalized for 8 days. He was breastfed for 15 days, with supplementation to maintain nutrition. There was no complaint regarding food and sleep. Regarding neuropsychomotor development, Hugo had presented cervical balance at 3 months, had sat with support at 5 months, without support at 7 months, crawled at 10 months, walked at 16 months, but still had not spoken a word at 23 months.

His parents reported that Hugo stayed at home with the mother, he did not attend school, and his screen time exposure during the day was very extensive (more than 5 hrs a day). At around 22 months of age, they began to reduce his exposure to screens, and Hugo began to babble sounds. His parents reported that Hugo did not point, did not carry out simple orders (in response to a command associated with a gesture), and used crying as the only means of communication. They also reported little eye contact, no play, and no response when Hugo was called by the name. The interaction improved after reducing the exposure to the screens. They also reported that when they left home, Hugo used to cover his ears with his hands until he adapted to environmental sounds, demonstrating auditory hypersensitivity; he did not play with other children and did not sit. He just liked to run and play ball. Hugo's family was referred with a diagnosis of ASD. Information about this condition is presented in the following section.

Check Your Progress

- What were Hugo's parents' main concerns about his development?

The Condition

ASD was first described in the literature by Austrian child psychiatrist Leo Kanner as *autistic disturbances of affective contact* (Kanner, 1943; Klin, 2006). In the *Diagnostic and Statistical Manual of Mental Disorders*, 5th edition (DSM-5; American Psychiatric Association, 2013), ASD is classified as a neurodevelopmental disorder characterized by persistent changes in the development of social (social reciprocity, maintenance, understanding of relationships) and linguistic skills (use of nonverbal language for interaction) and the presence of restricted and repetitive behaviors. First signs are usually seen before 3 years of age (chronological age), and its prevalence is higher in boys.

There is a constant growth in the knowledge of the characteristics of ASD (Yoon et al., 2020), as well as its multifactorial etiologies (genetic, epigenetic, and environmental factors). The development of resources such as intervention models, exams, and specific medications is ongoing, in addition to the practices of interdisciplinary monitoring and therapeutic procedures.

Regarding language development, which is one of the pillars of attention within ASD, studies of different natures (observational, meta-analyses, literature reviews), have shown the importance of observing the interaction and stimulus coming from the family, at early ages. The relationship with the rhythm and skills of language development is important (Edmunds et al., 2019; Fusaroli et al., 2019; Swanson et al., 2019). Olliac and colleagues (2017) have shown that early intervention can reduce delays and improve developmental outcomes for a significant proportion of children, and is able to reverse even secondary processes. This consideration reinforces the need for family guidance regarding directions and clarification on the importance of playing and stimulating children in their daily lives early on (Edmunds et al., 2019; Oono et al., 2013). Authors also emphasize the need to monitor parents' stress levels (Oono et al., 2013). A study related the parents' educational level to the language development of children with and without a diagnosis of ASD and found a direct relationship between these factors (Swanson et al., 2019).

A cross-sectional study in an Italian population sample found the first evident signs of ASD from between 7 and 12 months (41.9%) and between 13 and 24 months (27.6%) of chronological age, with 93.3% of cases relating to interaction and relationships and 92.4% to language development. Delay in oral language (speech) was one of the most common signs that led to an initial consultation for a possible diagnosis of ASD (Parmeggiani et al., 2019).

The Griffiths Scales of Child Development are an instrument used, among other things, to assess children with a suspected or confirmed diagnosis of ASD (Li et al., 2019; Li et al., 2020), and Griffiths III in its entirety has been translated and cross-culturally adapted (Ferreira-Vasques et al., 2019) and standardized for the Brazilian population of children from 0 to 24 months of age (Ferreira-Vasques, 2017).

Check Your Progress

- What can early intervention in language development support in a child with ASD?
- What aspects of family life should be considered?

The Consultation

Hugo, as reported, was a Brazilian 23-month-old boy with a diagnosis of ASD. In total, four sessions of speech therapy assessment were conducted and, in addition to the Observation of Communicative Behavior (Halle & Meaden, 2007), both the Denver-II Development Screening Test (Frankenburg & Archer, 1992) and the Griffiths III Scales of Child Development were administered.

During the first session, in which data about his history were collected with the help of his parents, Hugo was present and was free to do what he liked in the speech therapist's room. Connector blocks, formboards, and miniature toys such as carts, animals, food, and balls, in addition to paper and pencils, among other things were all available. In this first meeting, it was important for the parents to be present so that the child started his contact with the environment gradually, as well as so a rapport was developed, respecting the child's time. Parents were invited to remain in the assessment environment and instructed not to interfere during the application of the assessment instruments.

The Protocol for Observation of Communicative Behavior was completed, and a physical approach with the evaluator was verified, but not always with the intention of establishing communication. Hugo showed no initiative to interact, and when he wanted to leave the room, he cried and walked in the direction of the door. He accepted the offered toys and reproduced some movements, through imitation, in a restricted way. In a few moments, he presented brief eye contact, especially when called by the name.

His attention span was reduced, changing his object of interest several times, with superficial exploration and without assigning function or symbolic play. When Hugo had an object in his hand, he looked at it and then threw it on the floor. He showed some interest in the noise that the objects made when hitting the floor.

Hugo did not produce spoken words, nor did he use gestures, indicative or representative, to communicate. Crying and body movement were the only manifestations of communication. The last evaluation session, held in the morning, showed a difference in his performance and involvement, with better responses.

His interest in imitation was restricted, both during play, in games such as clapping hands, and in saying goodbye. He did not point out body parts or objects. His interest in pencils was summed up in playing and lining up, not using them to draw or doodle.

The result of the Denver-II Development Screening Test suggested that he was at risk of developmental delay. Using Hugo's chronological age of 23 months, the authors of this chapter developed a qualitative analysis of his skills as assessed in Denver-II. A new line of performance was drawn in each evaluated area, considering the skills he passed (performed) and those he failed (did not perform). This line of performance showed his skills to be compatible with children aged 21 months in the gross motor area, 15 months in fine adaptive motor control, 10 months in language, and 9 months in the personal-social area.

Hugo did not indicate his wants, wave bye bye, play ball, imitate activities, help in the house, use a spoon or fork, remove his garments, put on clothing, put on his shoes, build a tower with blocks, doodle vigorously, vocalize combined syllables, say dada or mama, speak isolated words or combine them, point to objects or figures, or kick a ball.

The Brazilian version of Griffiths III was also applied. Hugo's performance ages were below those expected for his chronological age (23 months), in all areas of child development. In general, Hugo performed better on Subscale E tasks (gross motor), comparable to Brazilian children aged 22 months; followed by Subscales A, C, and D, comparable to Brazilian children aged 15 months. In the Subscale B (language and communication), his performance was close to that of Brazilian children aged 10 months. Figures 7.1 and 7.2 above show the distribution of items achieved.

The Griffiths III base rate tables showed statistically significant differences between Hugo's scores on the Subscales A, B, C, and E. The Griffiths III base rate criteria confirmed that the magnitude of the dispersion indicated that the general development quotient was insufficient to describe all of Hugo's skills. It was important to compare the different analyses of the findings of the Griffiths Scales with the evaluations of other professionals involved in Hugo's care, as well as school and family reports.

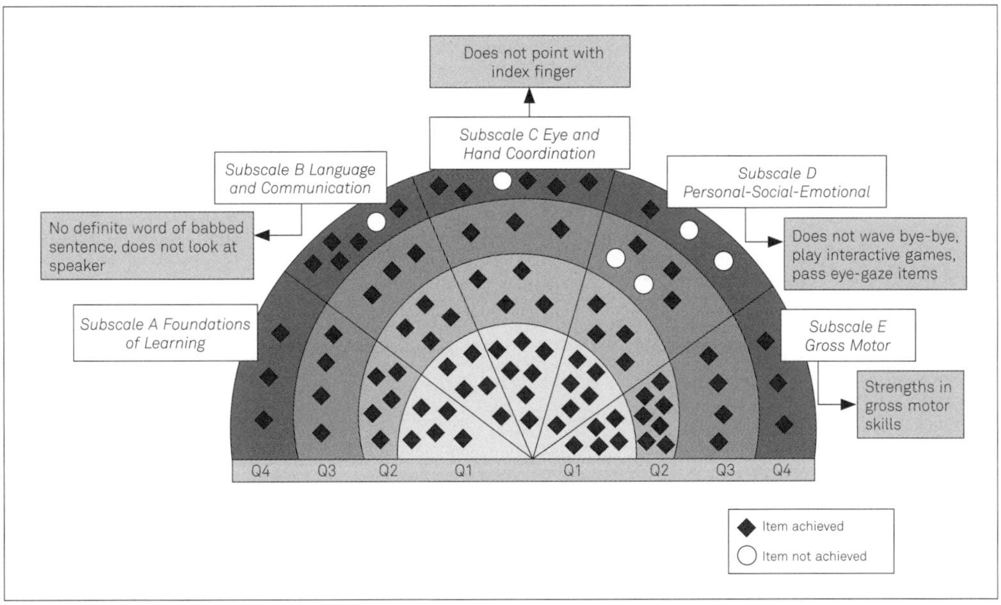

Figure 7.1. Distribution of items achieved or not achieved using the Griffiths III Quartile Chart Year 1. Q1 = Quartile level 1, achieved by 76–100% of typically developed children by year age; Q2 = Quartile level 2, achieved by 51–75% of typically developed children by year age; Q3 = Quartile level 3, achieved by 26–50% of typically developed children by year age; Q4 = Quartile level 4, achieved by 1–25% of typically developed children by year age

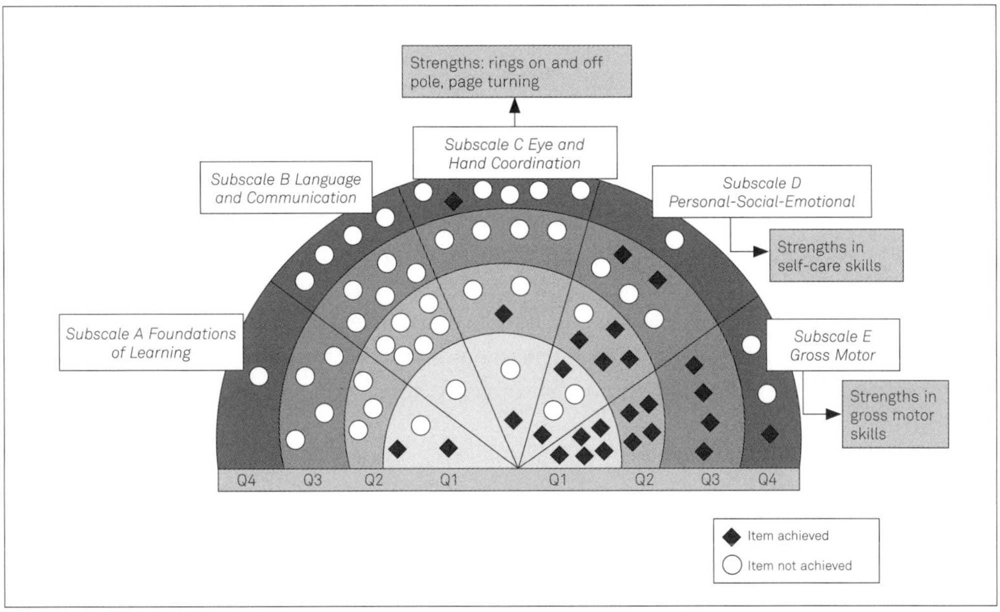

Figure 7.2. Distribution of items achieved or not achieved using the Griffiths III Quartile Chart Year 2. Q1 = Quartile level 1, achieved by 76–100% of typically developed children by year age; Q2 = Quartile level 2, achieved by 51–75% of typically developed children by year age; Q3 = Quartile level 3, achieved by 26–50% of typically developed children by year age; Q4 = Quartile level 4, achieved by 1–25% of typically developed children by year age

Check Your Progress

- Why were several assessments used?
- What were Hugo's main strengths and needs?

Connecting the Dots

When assessing a 23-month-old child, it is essential to hear the family's report of the child's life history, from its conception to the present moment. An authentic assessment looks closely at the family and reports from other professionals, and associates these with the observation and assessment of the child in the clinical environment, with the use of assessment instruments with constructs appropriate to the child's profile, to make a speech therapy diagnosis.

It is crucial to use standardized assessment instruments for the population in question, considering their cultural specificities, maintaining cross-cultural equivalences directly related to the construct of the material. The application of the Brazilian version of Griffiths III was fundamental to the diagnosis of developmental issues, linked with the observation of communicative behavior and family reporting, crucial for therapeutic planning, since the skills for each subscale evaluated in this instrument are placed in increasing order of difficulty and acquisition.

Another factor to be highlighted is knowledge of the child's routine as well as their functioning. Hugo performed better in the morning, and this was a finding that had not been observed by the family before the assessment. When school attendance began, the morning period was going to be the most suitable, specifically in the case of Hugo, as he would be more willing and receptive to stimuli and regulations. Therapies should also occur at times when the child is willing, for better assimilation of stimuli, acquisition of skills, and development of abilities.

Considering the clinical diagnosis of ASD and a general developmental disorder, with great damage to the language area, speech therapy was indicated, twice a week, with a direct weekly orientation session with the family. Evaluation by an occupational therapist was necessary also, to work on Hugo's sensory integration and admission to school. These procedures are based on knowledge about the importance of family orientation and their involvement in cases of children with early diagnosis of ASD, as well as the pace of evolution when the child is assisted by an interdisciplinary team that works in an integrated manner with child development.

Specifically, regarding the use of the Griffiths III Scales of Child Development to assess the development of Hugo, application of the items was easy, with continuity in the presentation of the items, with materials that are appropriate to the child population, even with that primary diagnosis of a neurodevelopmental disorder. The scales allow for an outline of a panorama of child development, respecting biopsychosocial and environmental aspects.

In ASD, communicative changes are very prevalent. The important changes in the language and communication subscale results for Hugo were confirmed by base rate analysis. The qualitative analysis of the items within the subscale directly assisted with the therapeutic planning for language stimulation.

Charting a Plan

The intervention plan formulated considered the family report with the results of the clinical and instrumentalized speech therapy assessment. Based on the knowledge of normative child development and its course and considering the interference that one area of development can inflict another, and vice versa, the planning was designed to stimulate absent skills with the use of present skills (strengths) as an anchor for the development to occur in a consistent and granular manner. The intervention plan includes family orientation, direct intervention, and orientations in school. These are described in the next sections.

Family Orientation

Various family orientation interventions are needed, including the following:

- The need for a reduction, aiming at its extinction, in Hugo's time spent in front of screens of any nature. In this way, Hugo will be available to perceive the environment and observe it, so that he can interact with it.
- School admission, since Hugo needs to spend time with his peers.
- Addressing the different means of communication that Hugo must and can use, in addition to crying and body movements, before he starts speaking.
- Clarifying the importance of eye contact, shared attention, pointing, and communicative exchange, with responses and actions to commands received, and maintaining the stimulus and motivation in activities of daily living in the family environment.
- Guidance regarding important toys to be made available, such as formboards and miniatures representing real objects from different semantic categories (animals, food, people, household items, means of transport, etc.), in addition to daily reading of age-appropriate books and playing with different textures and materials for drawing and coloring.
- Support for activities of daily living, allowing and encouraging autonomy in tasks consistent with Hugo's level of development (putting away toys, putting out water and food for the dog, throwing a diaper in the basket, eating on his own, and undressing).
- Guidance regarding and preparation of a supplementary and alternative communication portfolio, with real images of Hugo's toys and photos of his closest family members, as well as of the child himself, of foods of interest, and moments of daily routine, such as bathing, eating, and sleeping. The portfolio will also be used to encourage pointing, choosing, identifying, and answering questions (e.g., Where is the ball?).

Direct Intervention

Considering the skills not performed by Hugo in the administration of Griffiths III, it is possible to outline specific objectives, in sequence, using the predicted developmental milestones.

Besides making the supplementary augmentative and alternative communication portfolio, which is to be used with Hugo in speech therapy sessions, and for later guidance for the family and school regarding its use, it is important that the use of augmentative and alternative communication involves a consensus between the professional and the family. In this, the professional clarifies the importance and the gains to be achieved with the making and use of the portfolio, and, after the family understands and accepts this, the assembly process begins. Guidance for the family and school staff on how to use it is carried out constantly.

Skills such as pointing, recognizing objects, exploring toys and the environment in more elaborate ways, eye contact, communicative intention, and interaction with others, will be stimulated during sessions with Hugo, always analyzing their evolution, to expand and follow with more elaborate stimuli, such as symbolic play, gesture games, and peer games.

Gradually, new knowledge and means of communication are to be presented and stimulated so that Hugo develops his linguistic and communicative skills as well as those of other areas of development.

Orientation Toward School

This is extremely important. The teacher, the school team, and Hugo's classroom assistant should attend. This is to receive guidance, directly from the professional on a school visit, to learn about Hugo's current development and understand the stimulations and necessary adaptations in the school context. The communication portfolio, as well as visual routine, are crucial items to be addressed in this meeting, as they will permeate Hugo's communication and adjustment with adults and children living in the school environment.

Check Your Progress

- What information was the intervention plan based on?
- Why was the plan focused on different locations?

Conclusion

The main concepts presented in this chapter emphasize the importance of observing and assessing the child's global development, regardless of their diagnosis or condition. The family's report and the application of valid, standardized, and normalized assessment instruments, associated with professional experience and knowledge about child normative development, are indispensable factors for good management of the case. We also emphasize the importance of periodic reevaluations, using the same assessment instruments, to ensure the observation of the child's evolution.

Discussion Questions

- What are the interfering factors in the evaluation process of a child with ASD?
- How do you receive a family that has recently received a diagnosis of ASD for their child?
- What items should be considered in the therapeutic planning of a child with ASD? Reflect on the importance of different analyses of the results of the application of the Griffiths Scales, for adequate therapeutic planning.
- What is the importance of interdisciplinary assessment in ASD?
- What criteria should be used to decide which professionals are indicated to assess and monitor the longitudinal development of a child with ASD?

References

American Psychiatric Association. (2013). *Diagnostic and statistical manual of mental disorders* (5th ed.).

Edmunds, A. R., Kover, S. T., & Stone, W. L. (2019). The relation between parent verbal responsiveness and child communication in young children with oral risk for autism spectrum disorder: A systematic review and meta-analysis. *Autism Research, 12*(5), 715–731. https://doi.org/10.1002/aur.2100

Ferreira-Vasques, A. T. (2017). *Escala de desenvolvimento mental de Griffiths para crianças de 0 a 2 anos – adaptação para a população brasileira* [Griffiths mental development scale for children aged 0 to 2 years – Adaptation for the Brazilian population] [Unpublished doctoral dissertation]. Faculdade de Odontologia de Bauru, Universidade de São Paulo, Bauru.

Ferreira-Vasques, A. T., Santos, C. F., & Lamônica, D. A. C. (2019). Transcultural adaptation process of the Griffiths-III Mental Development Scale. *Child: Care, Health and Development, 45*(3), 403–408. https://doi.org/10.1111/cch.12664

Frankenburg, W. K., & Archer, P. (1992). *Denver II: Training manual* (2nd ed.). Denver Developmental Materials.

Fusaroli, R., Weed, E., Fein, D., & Naigles, L. (2019). Hearing me hearing you: reciprocal effects between child and parent language in autism and typical development. *Cognition, 183,* 1–18. https://doi.org/10.1016/j.cognition.2018.10.022

Halle, J., & Meaden, H. (2007). A protocol for assessing early communication of young children with autism and other developmental disabilities. *Topics in Early Childhood Special Education, 27*(1), 49–61. https://doi.org/10.1177/02711214070270010401

Kanner, L. (1943). Autistic disturbances of affective contact. *Nervous Child, 2*, 217–250.

Klin, A. (2006). Autismo e Síndrome de Asperger: Uma visão geral [Autism and Asperger syndrome: An overview]. *Brazilian Journal of Psychiatry, 28,* S3–S11. https://doi.org/10.1590/S1516-44462006000500002

Li, H.-H., Feng, J.-Y., Wang, B., Zhang, Y., Wang, C.-X., & Jia, F.-Y. (2019). Comparison of the children neuropsychological and behavior scale and the Griffiths Mental Development Scales when assessing the development of children with autism. *Psychology Research and Behavior Management, 16*(12), 973–981. https://doi.org/10.2147/PRBM.S225904

Li, P.-Y., Fu, N.-N., Li, Q.-Y., Wang, G.-F., Gao, L., & Zhang, X. (2020). The Griffiths Development Scales-Chinese (GDS-C): A reliable and valid neurodevelopmental assessment tool in children with ASD aged 3–8 years old in Tianjin, China. *Asian Journal of Psychiatry, 52,* 102144. https://doi.org/10.1016/j.ajp.2020.102144

Olliac, B., Crespin, G., Laznik, M. C., Ganouni, O. C. I., Sarradet, J. L., Bauby, C., Dandres, A. M., Ruiz, E., Bursztejn, C., Xavier, J., Falissard, B., Bodeau, N., Cohen, D., & Saint-Georges, C. (2017). Infant and dyadic assessment in early community-based screening for autism spectrum disorders with the PREAUT grid. *PLoS One, 12*(12): e0188831. https://doi.org/10.1371/journal.pone.0188831

Oono, I. P., Honey, E. J., & McConachie, H. (2013). Parent-mediated early intervention for young children with autism spectrum disorders (ASD). *Cochrane Database of Systematic Reviews, 30*(4), CD009774.

Parmeggiani, A., Corinaldesi, A., & Posar, A. (2019). Early features of autism spectrum disorder: A cross-sectional study. *Italian Journal of Pediatrics*, *45*(1), 144. https://doi.org/10.1186/s13052-019-0733-8

Swanson, M. R., Donovan, K., Paterson, S., Wolff, J. J., Parish-Morris, J., Meera, S. S., Watson, L. R., Estes, A. M., Marrus, N., Elison, J. T., Mark, D. S., McNeilly, H. B., Maclntyre, L., Zwaigenbaum, L., John, T. S., Botteron, K., Dager, S., Piven, J., & Network, I. (2019). Early language exposure supports later language skills in infants with and without autism. *Autism Research, 12*(12), 1784–1795.

Yoon, S. H., Choi, J., Lee, W. J., & Do, J. T. (2020). Genetic and epigenetic etiology: underlying autism spectrum disorder. *Journal of Clinical Medicine, 9*(4), 966. https://doi.org/10.3390/jcm9040966

Chapter 8

Jamie: Assessing a Child With High Functioning Autism

Ruth Paradice

The Context

Until I retired in 2019, I was a neurodevelopmental psychologist working in a local children's center in Wales in the UK. Children who came to the center were referred because of developmental delay. They would receive a multidisciplinary assessment from a team consisting of pediatricians, psychologists, speech and language therapists, occupational therapists, and physiotherapists. This assessment sometimes led to a diagnosis, but all children, regardless of diagnosis, received a detailed report outlining their strengths and needs and recommendations to support their development. My role was to carry out developmental assessments with a view to providing information for the team and recommendations for education.

The Child

Jamie was 3 years 4 months old when he was referred for a developmental assessment. He had already received a diagnosis of *autism spectrum disorder* (ASD), but it was not clear whether he had a learning disability in addition to this.

Jamie's parents were both working professionals. His father, Steve, had a PhD and worked in a scientific field, and Claire, his mother, was a secondary school teacher. There was no family history of neurodevelopmental difficulties.

Jamie's parents were concerned about aspects of his behavior and learning, which had come to light since starting nursery at the age of 3 years 1 month. The teaching staff reported that Jamie appeared aloof from the other children – he enjoyed playing alone and became very upset if other children attempted to join in with his play. Jamie's language was reported to be delayed for his age – he found it difficult to follow instructions and would not comply with classroom routines.

Jamie's parents felt he was very bright. They reported that he knew his alphabet, that he loved puzzles, and that he was "obsessed" with numbers. However, although advanced in some ways (he knew the names of a whole range of dinosaurs), Jamie's language had been slow to develop. He had not used single words consistently until he was about 20 months old. After that single words came quickly, and Jamie also repeated whole phrases that he had learned from the television programs and films that he liked to watch, but he did not always use these phrases in the right context, and he did not always understand instructions. He had been assessed by speech and language therapists. Their report indicated that Jamie's language was somewhat delayed, but they also noted that he struggled to follow adult direction and that his attention and listening skills were poor for activities that were not self-chosen.

Jamie's parents were still trying to toilet train him. Sleep was also an issue for him. It took him a long time to settle to sleep, and he woke very early in the morning, sometimes only getting around 5 hrs of sleep a night. Jamie was very fussy about food – he liked a very bland diet and wanted to eat the same thing over and over again. He was also very specific about which brands of crisps and yogurts he would eat, and he became extremely upset if his favorite brands were not available.

Check Your Progress

- What was the reason for Jamie's referral?
- What were his speech and language difficulties?

The Condition

ASD is a well-known condition in adults and children and is now recognized throughout the world, although it was not always so. It was first identified by Leo Kanner (1943/1968; quoted in Volmar et al., 2008), who described a syndrome which he called *early infantile autism*, which he believed to be a congenital disorder. This concurs with current thinking; there is now a lot of evidence to suggest that the basis of ASD is genetic. At about the same time, Asperger (1944; quoted in Barahon-Correa & Filipe, 2015) identified a slightly different group of children who shared many of the features of the group noted by Kanner, with the exception that they did not suffer from learning difficulties and were thus what we now call *high functioning.*

ASD occurs in about 1% of children and young people (Kendal et al., 2013). It is a disability that is lifelong. There are big differences among individuals diagnosed with autism, but the core features are persistent impairment in reciprocal social interaction and social communication and restricted, repetitive patterns of behavior, interests, or activities. Individuals may or may not have a learning disability in addition. Those with average intelligence are described as high functioning.

According to the criteria outlined in the *Diagnostic and Statistical Manual of Mental Disorders,* 5th edition (DSM-5; American Psychiatric Association, 2013), a child must have persistent deficits in each of three areas of social communication and interaction, plus at least two of four types of restricted, repetitive behavior. These could include stereotyped or repetitive motor movements, insistence on sameness and inflexible adherence to routines, or highly restricted interests that are abnormal in intensity. Symptoms must be present in the early developmental period and must cause clinically significant impairment in social, occupational, or other important areas of functioning.

As there is no definitive test for ASD, all diagnoses are based on clinical judgment. Therefore, a detailed history and careful observation of the child in a range of different situations is essential.

Check Your Progress

- Do some children with ASD have average intelligence?

The Consultation

Jamie was initially reluctant to engage with the equipment presented and appeared very shy, but after a while his curiosity got the better of him, and he started to explore the brick boxes that had been laid out on the table. He coped best with the assessment if I did not look at him directly and minimized my use of language as much as possible. Once he became interested in a task, it was difficult to move him on to something else, and there were certain tasks that he refused completely.

Subscale A

Jamie completed the formboards very quickly, although it was difficult to get him to wait while the pieces were being stacked. It was not clear whether he really understood the instruction to try to complete the formboards "even faster" on the second trial.

Jamie assembled the brick boxes by color, but he could not build a bridge or a castle. This did not appear to be due to a lack of ability, but he found it hard to follow adult direction and wanted to put the bricks and the boxes together in this own way. This was also a problem with the memory house task. This was exacerbated by the more complex instructions for this task, which was also an issue with the series tasks. Jamie's issues with understanding complex instructions and following adult direction meant that he could not complete many of the tasks in the Year 4 section of the test in this subscale.

Subscale B

Jamie was good at naming objects – he could correctly identify all 16 objects in the box and give all the names of the objects depicted in the picture vocabulary. He was able to name the six verbs in the activity pictures and in fact could manage all eight, but I could not score him for this because he had failed the previous six items. Jamie could name a lot of the objects in the large picture, but he could not make up a story from the picture. Some of the words he used to describe objects in the large picture seemed rather sophisticated for his age. Jamie talked well in sentences using five and more words; for example, he told me, "I didn't go to nursery today," but he did not always answer questions, and if we look at the items he passed in this subscale, it was notable that his expressive language was better developed than his receptive language. This is a somewhat unusual pattern, as generally a child's comprehension of language (receptive language) will be more advanced than their use of language (expressive language). This was highlighted in Jamie's difficulties with following instructions, defining objects by use, and understanding opposites and similarities.

Subscale C

Jamie could put the connector blocks together – but it was difficult to move him on from this task. His mother commented that he loved playing with connector blocks at home and would spend hours with this, so he wanted to continue playing with them. Fortunately, Jamie was quite interested in the bead-threading task, and he was happy to thread the beads onto the string. He managed 11+ beads with ease. Jamie was also able to copy a horizontal stroke, but could only manage a very wobbly circle which was not good enough to pass, I noticed during this activity that his pencil grasp was quite weak. He refused to touch the playdough – he clearly did not like the feel of it, and while we were attempting this task, his mother explained that there were quite a number of textures that Jamie did not like. In nursery he would play in the water but would not go near the sand pit. I could not get him interested in undoing the buttons.

Subscale D

This proved to be the most difficult subscale for Jamie – he was able to tell me his first name when I asked him and he could say his age – he also knew that he was a boy, but he was unable to give his family name. He could identify "happy" and "sad" on the facial expressions cards, but I could not score him for dressing, as his mother told me that dressing was a real battle every morning, and he refused to help with this. He had a few items of clothing that he wanted to wear all of the time, and unless he could wear these, he would not cooperate with dressing at all.

Jamie was not able to express his own thoughts and feelings, he was struggling with toilet training and would not participate in group play. He did not seem to understand the perspective-taking cards at all, and his mother reported that he did not appear to notice if she, or another person was hurt or upset.

Subscale E

Jamie was able to jump off a step – he was quick walking upstairs, and he could rise from kneeling without using his hands. I could not score him for running fast, because although he did run, it was not fast and looked somewhat awkward. I did not observe smooth and regular alternating strides. I could not score him for crossing feet and knees when seated because he would not copy me, although I did manage to get him to stand on one foot for 3 seconds. Jamie could not catch a tennis ball, and he would not attempt the activities involving tapes, so he might have been able to do these if he had complied.

Check Your Progress

- How was Jamie helped to participate in the consultation?
- Was his receptive or expressive language more developed?

Connecting the Dots

Jamie was 3 years 4 months old with an existing diagnosis of ASD, but it was not clear whether he had a learning disability in addition to this. Jamie's parents and teaching staff at his nursery were concerned about aspects of his behavior and learning. Concerns related to aloof behavior, distress if other children attempted to join him, delayed language development, difficulty following instructions, and lack of compliance with classroom routines. Jamie's parents felt he was very bright with some achievements such as knowing his alphabet and puzzles; also that he was "obsessed" with numbers. His language development had been slow. Other issues at home were toilet training, sleep and fussiness about food. Table 8.1 below shows Jamie's results obtained on the Griffiths III assessment.

Table 8.1. Jamie's results on Griffiths III assessment

Subscale	Raw score	Developmental age (months)	Scaled score	Development quotient	Percentile
Subscale A	37	34	8	87	20
Subscale B	39	31	5	76	7
Subscale C	40	32	6	80	10
Subscale D	33	24	1	52	< 1
Subscale E	39	31	5	73	5
General development	37.6	30	4	68	3

Jamie's scaled scores ranged from 8 to 1, showing an interscale scatter of 7 points. The base rates from the standardization sample indicated that this was not statistically significant; 17.1% of children in the standardization sample also showed this level of difference between subscales. Therefore, it was appropriate to calculate the general development (GD) score, which was 68.

The GD score alone, however, does not give a very clear picture of Jamie's strengths and needs. To get a more nuanced picture of his developmental profile, it was more helpful to look at individual subscales, as this showed areas where Jamie was doing well and areas where he needed more support. A comparison of Jamie's scores across the subscales using the discrepancy tables showed where there were significant differences between subscales and the GD. Please note that anything that occurs in less than 10% of the standardization sample is to be regarded as statistically significant. Table 8.2 below shows the significant differences between the subscales of the Griffiths III assessment.

Table 8.2. Significant (Sig) vs. nonsignificant (NS) differences for Jamie between subscale scores

Discrepancy	A vs. B	A vs. C	A vs. D	A vs. E	B vs. C	B vs. D	B vs. E	C vs. D	C vs. E	D vs. E
Difference in scores	+3	+2	+7	+3	-1	+4	0	+5	+1	-4
% Base rate	15.6	32.8	0.0	25.0	32.8	9.4		7.8	50.0	9.4
Significance	NS	NS	Sig	NS	NS	Sig	NS	Sig	NS	Sig

Table 8.2 shows significant differences between subscales A and D, B and D, C and D, and D and E. Subscale D seems to be the common denominator, which is consistent with Jamie's diagnosis of autism.

We can also compare Jamie's scores on each of the subscales with his score on the GD scale. These results are shown in Table 8.3.

Table 8.3. Significant (Sig) vs. nonsignificant (NS) differences for Jamie between subscale scores and general development (GD)

Discrepancy	A vs. GD	B vs. GD	C vs. GD	D vs. GD	E vs. GD
Difference in scores	+4	+1	+2	-3	+1
% Base rate	1.6	50.0	12.5	12.5	32.8
Significance	Sig	NS	NS	NS	NS

In Table 8.3, we see that although there was a significant difference between Subscale A and GD, none of the other comparisons reach significance.

Strengths

- The results for Subscale A indicated that Jamie was a little boy who was of at least average intelligence. His development quotient of 87 was probably an underestimation of his ability, because there were some items that he refused to engage with, and others where his difficulties with receptive language meant that he did not always understand the task.

- Jamie was really good at naming things, and he had a good vocabulary for his age. His expressive language was a strength.
- Jamie loved puzzles and was good at solving them.
- He had very good concentration on things that interested him.

Needs

- Jamie struggled to follow adult direction.
- His understanding of language was not so good and might be masked by his expressive language. Jamie's low score on Subscale B highlighted this. An analysis of the constructs underpinning the failed items in this subscale indicated that receptive language was an area in which Jamie needed some additional help.
- His sensory difficulties meant that there were some things that he found hard to engage with. Jamie's scores on Subscale C were just about in the average range. This score would have been higher if he had not had sensory difficulties, which meant that he would not handle the playdough.
- He struggled with engaging with adults and children, he preferred to do things his own way. Subscale D was an area that clearly highlighted Jamie's difficulties with social engagement, and this subscale stood out in the statistical analysis, differing significantly from his scores on all of the other subscales. He could not be scored for playing with other children and having a playmate. He was unable to dress or undress himself. He was struggling with toilet training, and he could not take the perspective of another. He also lacked empathy and did not respond to the emotions of others, although he was starting to recognize facial expressions.

Check Your Progress

- Why was Jamie's DQ felt to be an underestimate?
- How was the significance of the subscale scores calculated?

Charting a Plan

Jamie's profile on Griffiths III, taken together with his presentation in clinic and information from his parents and his nursery school, was consistent with a child with high functioning ASD. He did not present as a child with a learning disability, although some of his issues with receptive language and his reluctance to engage with others might well have an impact on his learning over time.

Jamie should be able to cope in a mainstream setting, but he might need additional help to access the curriculum and develop social relationships with other children. He has quite specific interests in certain tasks which he focuses on to the exclusion of other learning opportunities, so he needs encouragement to engage with a range of different materials – perhaps using his passions to introduce new ideas and experiences.

Jamie's expressive language is better developed than his receptive language. We tend to assume that if a child can use language, they can also understand it, but in Jamie's case this is a dangerous assumption to make. Jamie struggles to follow instructions, and he could not always understand what was expected of him. Jamie's understanding of language needed to be supported by

- Not overwhelming him with too much language,
- Keeping language brief and to the point,
- Checking that he had understood what had been said, and
- Using visual cues to support his understanding.

A visual timetable would help Jamie to understand the school day and classroom routines. He should not be expected to sit for long periods of time listening to language-based activities. Such activities should be specifically tailored for him within a smaller group of children. It would be helpful to consult with a speech and language therapist for additional strategies to support Jamie's language.

Jamie would benefit from additional support in managing his sensory difficulties by slowly introducing textures that he dislikes, and using his interests is a useful strategy: for example, hiding his favorite connector blocks under playdough, in dry and wet pasta, or in shaving foam. His pencil grip is also quite weak, so activities to strengthen his hands would be beneficial. Advice from an occupational therapist could be sought for more specific and targeted strategies.

Jamie struggles to play with other children. He needs adult support to establish friendships. Perhaps he could be paired with one or two other children in small group activities to encourage sharing and turn taking. Perhaps it would be possible for his mother to invite another child home to play after nursery for a short time (30 minutes). Cooperative and social play do not come easily to Jamie, so it is important to devise situations where he has the opportunity to learn these skills from other children, but also from adults modeling sharing, turn taking, and cooperating. Finally, he needs to be encouraged to spend time in more physical outdoor play to assist the development of his gross motor skills.

Check Your Progress

- What support was suggested for Jamie's language?
- What support was suggested to manage his sensory difficulties?

Conclusion

This assessment has highlighted many of the difficulties of carrying out an authentic assessment of a child with autism. Children with ASD may find the testing situation stressful, and the nature of their difficulties means that they struggle to comply with adult-led activities. Nevertheless, the results obtained certainly supported the diagnosis of ASD and also demonstrated that Jamie did not have a learning difficulty in addition to ASD.

Discussion Questions

You may like to consider how you would adapt the testing situation to ensure that a child such as Jamie has the best opportunity to achieve their full potential. You may want to consider:

- The setting: Is a clinic room or other unfamiliar place the best environment? Would the child be better off being assessed in their home, or maybe at school? There are both advantages and disadvantages to using these environments, but they should be considered in the context of the individual you are planning to assess.
- The tasks: Are there ways of adapting the tasks so that the child finds them more engaging? You want to know what the child is able to do when given the best opportunity. However, you must be aware that if you change the task, you cannot score the test in a standardized way.
- The language: Can you find ways to minimize or simplify the language of the test? Again, if you change the language too much, then you cannot score the test in a standardized way, but you might be able to discover what adaptations are needed to enable the child to succeed at a particular task.
- What motivates the child? Can you use their passions to see what they can achieve? For example, Jamie loved dinosaurs and knew a lot about them, perhaps his interest could be used to adapt the tasks to show what he is capable of.

Finally, if you want to know more about autism a useful book is *Autism: A New Introduction to Psychological Theory and Current Debate* (Fletcher-Watson & Happé, 2019)

References

American Psychiatric Association. (2013). *Diagnostic and statistical manual of mental disorders* (5th ed.) https://doi.org/10.1176/appi.books.9780890425596

Asperger, H. (1944). Die "Autistischen Psychopathen" im Kindesalter [The "Autistic psychopaths" in childhood]. *Archiv für Psychiatrie und Nervenkrankheiten, 117,* 76–136. https://doi.org/10.1007/BF01837709

Barahon-Correa, J. B., & Filipe, C. N. (2015). A concise history of Asperger's syndrome: The short reign of a troublesome diagnosis. *Frontiers in Psychology, 6,* 2024–2026. https://doi.org/10.3389/fpsyg.2015.02024

Fletcher-Watson, S., & Happé, F. (2019). *A new introduction to psychological theory and current debate.* Routledge.

Kanner, L. (1968). Autistic disturbances of affective contact. *Acta Paedopsychiatica, 35,* 100–135. (Original work published 1943).

Kendal, T., Megnin-Viggars, O., Gould, N., Taylor, C., Burt, L. R., & Baird, G. (2013). Management of autism in children and young people: Summary of NICE and SCIE guidance. *British Medical Journal, 347,* 34–36. https://doi.org/10.1136/bmj.f4865

Volmar, F. R., Chawarska, K., & Kin, A. (2008). Autism spectrum disorders in infants and toddlers. In K. Charwarska, A. Klin, & F. R. Volmar (Eds.), *Autism spectrum disorders in infants and toddlers: Diagnosis, assessment and treatment.* Guilford Press.

Chapter 9

Eli: Assessing a Child With Low Functioning Autism

Ruth Paradice

The Context

As mentioned in Chapter 8, until I retired in 2019, I was a neurodevelopmental psychologist with a background in educational psychology, working in a local children's center in Wales in the UK. Children who came to the center were referred because of developmental delay. They would receive a multidisciplinary assessment from a team consisting of pediatricians, psychologists, speech and language therapists, occupational therapists, and physiotherapists. This assessment sometimes led to a diagnosis, but all children, regardless of diagnosis, received a detailed report outlining their strengths and needs and recommendations to support their development. My role was to carry out developmental assessments with a view to providing information for the team and recommendations for education.

The Child

Eli was 3 years 2 months old when he was referred for a developmental assessment. The pediatricians who had seen Eli were confident that he was showing signs of autism, but they had requested a developmental assessment to decide whether in addition he had a learning disability.

Eli's parents were living in the UK as asylum seekers. His mother spoke very little English, and she did not work but stayed at home looking after Eli. Eli's father was making his living driving a taxi. His English was better, and he was hoping to do further training once he knew that the family could settle in the UK. Eli's parents had no support from extended family, as they had fled their home country leaving everything and everyone behind them. They were keen to speak in English to Eli and were concerned that speaking two languages to him had caused his speech and language difficulties. We explained to them that this was not the case, and it was better to speak to him in their mother tongue, rather than in a language that they were still learning themselves, as this gave him a better model of language.

Eli's parents first became concerned about him when he failed to start talking. He was their first child, so they had no experience of typical child development. However, they did expect that he would have started saying his first words at around 12 months. In fact, they did feel that he knew some words at this age; they thought that he had said "Dada" and

"Mumma," but at 18 months, these word-like sounds had disappeared. Eli did make vocalizations, but these largely consisted of shouts and screams, and they did not appear to be directed at other people. When asked about his early history, they described a very "good" baby who initially had made very few demands. As he got older, however, they had noticed that he was often quite difficult to soothe when he became distressed. He did not appear to enjoy being cuddled, and he did not make eye contact with them. He smiled rather late, and although he smiled quite a lot, it was not a social smile – that is, he smiled to himself, but he did not respond with a smile when someone else smiled at him.

Eli was physically very active. At home he liked to run around the house, and he particularly liked to climb up on furniture. This could be quite dangerous, as he liked to climb as high as possible, and he would try to climb up onto the kitchen units and also onto bookcases. Parents had put locks on many of the doors; they were particularly concerned that he would run out through the front door. He had no awareness of traffic, and they lived on quite a busy road.

At home Eli liked to watch TV, and his parents often used this to calm him down and to keep him quiet, because if the TV was not on, he would simply keep running around the house. Eli loved light switches and was constantly flicking them on and off. He also liked to look at lights and would stare fixedly at them, sometimes looking from unusual angles. Eli also enjoyed flicking paper in front of his face and looking at his hands. He would often run around with his hands in front of him – not looking at where he was going but watching his hands spread out in front of him.

Eli was not yet toilet trained and had no awareness of having wet or soiled his nappy. His parents had not attempted to toilet train him. He slept well but would not sleep in his own bed, he shared a bed with his mother. He ate a very restricted diet. He would use his fingers to eat some foods, but otherwise his mother fed him. He would not sit at a table, but his parents were so concerned about his food intake that they followed him around the house, trying to get him to eat.

When I met with Eli initially and before attempting any kind of assessment, I quickly appreciated that it would be difficult to carry out an assessment using Griffiths III in a standardized way.

Check Your Progress

- What were the family's concerns about Eli?
- What role does the family's restricted use of English play and how should this be managed?

The Condition

Autism spectrum disorder (ASD) has already been briefly described in Chapter 8. In that section it was noted that children with autism could have average levels of intelligence but could also have a learning disability. The *Diagnostic and Statistical Manual of Mental Disorders,* 5th edition (DSM-5; American Psychiatric Association, 2013) explicitly states that a diagnosis of autism can only be given if the 'symptoms' are not better explained by a learning disability, so although Eli was thought to have autism in addition to a learning disability it was important to clarify this.

In general terms the outcome for children with autism who also have learning difficulties is poorer. These children may well remain nonverbal throughout their lives and may also require greater levels of support. DSM-5 outlines three levels of support that might be needed by individuals. The highest level of need is Level 3 where individuals demonstrate severe deficits in communication skills both verbal and nonverbal, extreme difficulty in coping with change, extreme difficulty with shifting focus and attention, and demonstrate very limited amounts of social interaction.

Check Your Progress

- What are the three levels of support outlined by DSM-5?

The Consultation

On the day of the assessment I made sure that there were no distracting toys around the room other than the Griffiths III kit, but it was difficult to get Eli to focus on any of the equipment. He preferred to trot around the room, and he frequently went to the door and ran out into the corridor. He enjoyed running down the corridor. He did not respond to his mother calling his name, and she told me that this was how he behaved when they were outside, so she was always very anxious that he would run away from her or go off with a complete stranger. Eventually, with his mother's permission we had to lock the door of the clinic room to prevent Eli from opening it and running away.

Subscale A

Most of the items in the first year of this subscale were "scored" through observation and discussion with Eli's parents. So, I noted that he was able to pick up a brick from the table – he did glance at an object that fell to the floor. He passed a brick from hand to hand, and he could take the bricks out of the brick box. He was able to pull at a cloth to get a toy, but it took a long time to gain his attention for this task, and we had to find an object that was very high value, that was something that he really wanted. It was not possible to keep his attention long enough to see if he could manage the A not B task. The formboards were placed on the floor near to Eli, and I noted that he was able to put all of the shapes in. It was not possible to do any of the items for Year 3, because of Eli's poor attention span and also his very limited language.

Subscale B

Eli had no language at all. He made vocalizations, largely to himself, and he often shouted and shrieked. It was very difficult to establish a baseline for this subscale and to score it, we were dependent on Eli's parents telling us what they could remember of his infancy. They felt that he had babbled and that he had responded when called. He would respond to sounds, and he liked to look at books. Although Eli had no words at all, his parents told me that they thought he "understood everything." It was not possible to score any of the items for Year 2 of this subscale.

Subscale C

We were able to observe Eli putting the rings on the ring pole, but he could not be persuaded to build a tower of bricks – his parents told me that he would build with bigger building blocks at home. He would not hold a pencil or crayon, and so I was unable to assess whether he could make a circular scribble in imitation. Eli was interested in the connector blocks, and he did put those together. He also turned the pages of a book.

Subscale D

This was another subscale where it was impossible to establish a baseline. Once again we were very dependent on information from Eli's parents. His parents felt that Eli recognized them. He quite liked looking at his reflection in a mirror. They believed that he anticipated being picked up when he was small. He liked rhymes and jingles when he heard them on the TV. He would drink from a beaker, and in his own way he gave affection, although it was usually on his own terms – he did not like it if parents tried to cuddle him, but he was fine if he went to them for a cuddle. He liked to take his clothes off, and this was sometimes difficult as he liked to be without clothes when he was in the house and would frequently run around naked.

Subscale E

Eli was physically a very active little boy; he loved climbing and was very agile. He could run fast. He could squat to play on the floor. It was more difficult to assess whether he could walk backwards pulling a toy on a string, as I could not persuade him to do this. He was not interested in trying to throw a short tennis ball into a basket, and he was not interested in copying me crossing my legs and ankles. In this subscale there were several things that he might have been able to do had his language been better and had he had more interest in social interaction. Table 9.1 below shows Eli's results obtained on the Griffiths III assessment.

Eli's scaled scores range from 0 to 3 showing an interscale scatter of 3 points. If we look at the base rates from the standardization sample, we can see that this difference was not statistically significant. Therefore, it was appropriate to calculate the general development score.

Table 9.1. Eli's Griffiths III scores

Subscale	Raw score	Developmental age (months)	Scaled score	Development quotient	Percentile
Subscale A	23	19	0	50	1
Subscale B	10	20	0	< 50	< 1
Subscale C	26	20	0	< 50	< 1
Subscale D	16	20	0	< 50	< 1
Subscale E	35	27	3	62	1
General development	22	22	0	< 50	< 1

Although we calculated scores for each subscale and a general development score based on the above figures, this score alone did not give a very clear picture of Eli's strengths and needs, based as it was on a test that was not administered in a standardized way. It gave us only a broad picture of his abilities, which might, in fact, have been either an overestimation or underestimation. When a child's standard scores are as low as they were in Eli's case, it is helpful to look at the quartile charts, which give us a more detailed and nuanced picture that is relevant and helpful for making recommendations.

Check Your Progress

- Was it possible to estimate Eli's baseline for the subscales?
- How was the assessment scored?

Connecting the Dots

Subscale A

Eli was able to complete most of the items for Year 2, achieving what only 1–25% of children in Year 2 could manage. He passed no items for Year 3. The Griffiths III analysis based on scores alone suggested a developmental age of 19 months, but the quartile charts suggested that this was an underestimation, and his developmental age was probably nearer 24 months. We also noted that the items passed were primarily visual, suggesting that Eli would need materials presented visually to help to develop his learning.

Subscale B

Language and communication was an area of difficulty for Eli. Although he achieved a developmental age score of 20 months on the Griffiths III analysis, when we considered the quartile charts, this was probably an overestimation of his language ability. The items that he passed on this subscale were mainly those that would be passed by 26–50% of children in their first 12 months of life. He did not pass any items for Year 2 of this subscale, and so his ability was more in the 9- to 12-month age range.

Subscale C

Eli passed all items for Year 1 of the eye and hand coordination subscale, but his passes and fails became patchier after this, mainly because of his difficulties with social engagement and following instructions. He was able to manage one of the later items for Year 2 and one of the earlier items for Year 3. As with Subscale A, the results were a slight underestimation of the developmental age of his ability, which would probably have been more accurately reported as around 24 months.

Subscale D

Eli did relatively well on the self-help skills in this subscale. He was able to take his clothes off, although he did this inappropriately. He could manage a cup. Once again his language and social interaction problems meant that there were many items that he failed. His scores were scattered across the Year 2 level, so the quartile charts did not really help us to be more precise in this subscale.

Subscale E

The standard Griffiths III analysis for the gross motor subscale gave Eli a developmental age of 23 months. In fact, Eli passed the first four items for Year 3 – these would be achieved by most children in Year 3, and so it was likely that his gross motor skills were largely age appropriate. His lower score as calculated by the standard analysis was an underestimation of his true ability, caused by his difficulty in following instructions.

Check Your Progress

- Did the quartile charts give extra information about Eli's skills?

Charting a Plan

As Eli has ASD and a learning difficulty, he is likely to struggle in a mainstream setting unless he has some extra support to enable him to access learning opportunities and make progress. It could be that a specialist school with smaller class sizes and specialist teachers, might be the best option for him. Box 9.1 shows a summary of his strengths and needs.

Box 9.1. Eli's strengths and needs

Strengths
- Eli is a visual learner; he is good at puzzles
- His gross motor skills are largely age appropriate
- He has some good self-help skills – he can feed himself and take his clothes off
- His fine motor skills are also a relative strength

Needs
- Eli finds it hard to focus and follow adult direction
- He can not communicate his wants and needs
- He struggles to communicate with others
- He does not know how to make relationships with adults or children
- He is not yet toilet trained
- He has no awareness of danger

Eli's visual skills need to be harnessed to help him learn to communicate using Augmentative and Alternative Communication (AAC). At first, he needs to be helped to understand how a symbol can be used to communicate with others. The Picture Exchange Communication System (PECS), which was developed in the US in 1985, is a language program that is used extensively in the UK (Bondy & Frost, 1985). It uses picture symbols to enable children with little or no language to communicate. A system of traffic light symbols could also be used at home and at nursery to help Eli understand when an activity was to start (green symbol), when it was nearly finished (orange symbol), and when it was to stop (red symbol) - this should help him be less frustrated. A simple visual timetable could be developed to help him to understand when things would happen. Once he begins to learn that symbols have meanings that enable him to interpret what is happening in the world around him, his level of frustration should decrease and his concentration increase. Traffic lights should also help Eli stop doing things that are dangerous, such as climbing up on high furniture, running off when out in the street, etc.

Eli is good at undressing, but not so good at dressing. *Backward chaining* could be used to help him understand how to put clothes on, starting with simple things such as socks and jogging bottoms. The technique of *backward chaining* involves breaking a practical task down into its component parts to enable the child to achieve full mastery of the task. Let us consider the task of putting on a sock: by starting with the simplest part of the task, i.e., putting one's toes into the rolled down sock, the child can be encouraged to learn how to pull the sock up a little until eventually they are able to put the whole sock on. The same process can then be followed by other tasks.

Check Your Progress

- Why were Eli's visual skills used to support his developmental progress?
- Why was backward-chaining suggested?

Conclusion

This assessment highlighted many of the difficulties of carrying out an authentic assessment of a child whose scores fall below the 1st percentile. The quartile charts can help by giving us a more detailed perspective of the child's strengths and needs.

Discussion Questions

It may be helpful to look at the quartile charts and consider how you might use them yourself for a child whose score was below the 1st percentile. Consider:

- What would be the benefits? What are the disadvantages?
- Is a standardized test such as Griffiths III the best way of assessing a child like this? What other methods could you use to describe their needs?
- What is the parent's perspective likely to be? What aspects of the child's presentation will they be finding it most difficult to cope with? Are their priorities different from those of the clinical or educational context?
- If so, how can people work together to best help the child? What motivates the child?

Finally, if you want to know more about autism, a useful book is *Autism: A New Introduction to Psychological Theory and Current Debate* (Fletcher-Watson & Happé, 2019).

References

American Psychiatric Association. (2013). *Diagnostic and statistical manual of mental disorders* (5th ed.) https://doi.org/10.1176/appi.books.9780890425596

Bondy, A., & Frost, L. (1985). *Pecs® The Picture Exchange Communication System.* Pyramid Educational Products.

Fletcher-Watson, S., & Happé, F. (2019). *A new introduction to psychological theory and current debate.* Routledge.

Chapter 10

Victor: Resilience in the COVID-19 Pandemic

Iolanda Gil, Carlota Ferreira, Inês Carvalhão, and Solange Fernandes

The Context

The authors of this case study are a group of senior psychologists and Griffiths Scales tutors from Lisbon, Portugal, with work experience in complex neurodevelopmental disorders. Using a descriptive case study method, we assessed Victor (fictitious name to protect and maintain his anonymity) during psychological consultations in a child developmental department at a rehabilitation center. The purpose of this case study is to illustrate how important and useful the follow-up assessments with Griffiths Scales are for children, and to show the importance of their parents' resilience, in the context of the first lockdown in the COVID-19 pandemic. The case study also describes a high level of consistency between the profile used in both the Griffiths Scales, the Griffiths Mental Development Scales (GMDS-ER) in the first assessment, and Griffiths III in the second assessment.

The Child

Victor was a 6-year-old child. He lived with his parents, who had successfully achieved a university education at degree level, with established careers. They were able to provide financial stability and a healthy family environment to their child.

Even though Victor was attending preschool, his classes were interrupted by the 2020 pandemic lockdown, from March until August, while both parents were also working from home. This was his first preschool year, as he had been with his grandmother due to respiratory problems. During the lockdown period, Victor's parents had frequent online support from our professionals, to continue developing his special autonomy and motor skills, as well as language exercises using communication cards, music, and adapted story telling with pictographic systems.

In September 2020, Victor restarted attending preschool, and his teacher started reporting his constant avoidant behavior. This behavior was manifested toward other children as well as members of school staff. During his first month, as he restarted his routine, which included therapy sessions and preschool, his social interaction skills and verbal communication slowly emerged. Victor increased his vocabulary, by using isolated words, mostly in an echolalia form, with his team and adults. By December, he was communicating in simple two-word sentences, which was driven by the recent opportunity to play with his schoolmates. We could conclude that, within his first month of school, he was able to recover and improve his social skills with unfamiliar individuals. Finally, even though Victor's social skills with other children had suffered the negative impact of lockdown, he had significantly improved his language skills as a result of the different therapies and support provide to the family and his parents' support.

Victor was first and only child in a family with no history of any diseases. His parents were a healthy and nonconsanguineous young couple. He was born at term, with Apgar scores 10/10 and normal range weight, and his mother had had no intercurrent illnesses during pregnancy and childbirth. He had achieved normal milestones up to 12 months in gross and fine motor development and language skills.

The first symptoms of social interaction and communication with repetitive pattern behaviors that had a functional impact in language, including the loss of some words and sounds and avoidance of eye contact, began when he was 12 months old. Victor also started having frequent and severe respiratory infections, as well as otitis at this stage.

Medical Investigation Results

A neuronal examination, in the form of an electroencephalogram, brain magnetic resonance imaging, and spectroscopy, was normal. Auditory evocated potential was normal. The genetics investigation included arrayCGH/CytoSure Constitutional and molecular study for fragile X syndrome, and these were normal. Dysmorphic phenotype minor was present and waiting for exome research. Metabolic research was carried out for molecular trimethylaminuria and included in the FIND project.

Check Your Progress

- When did Victor start to have more contact with his parents?

The Condition

At that time, Victor had multiple diagnoses with comorbidities:

- Immunity disease, immunoglobulin A (IgA) deficit, with severe and repeated respiratory and urinary infections,
- Autism spectrum disorder (ASD), confirmed on the Childhood Autism Rating Scale (CARS) to be at a moderate/severe level,
- Autism phenotype of atypical sleep patterns, with prolonged and frequent nocturnal awakenings, and
- Developmental delays.

The signs of ASD emerge in the first 2 years of life, and are clinically and etiologically heterogeneous, characterized by social interaction and communication deficits and repetitive and stereotyped behavior (Baio et al., 2018; Rosenberg et al., 2009). Autism is not a single disorder but a neurodevelopmental syndrome and a widely variable spectrum of comorbidities (Geschwind, 2011).

Check Your Progress

- What were Victor's diagnoses?

The Consultation

First Assessment

Victor came to our psychology consultation with the purpose of an evaluation and intervention. Functional evaluations of development were carried out using clinical observation, the *International Classification of Functioning, Disability and Health of Children and Youth* (ICF-CY), and normative Griffiths Scales, to design an intervention plan. The functional assessment is made with the ICF-CY checklist (WHO, 2013) using the main concerns of parents and professional teams regarding Victor's functioning. Table 10.1 below shows his functional impairment in body functions, and mental functions related to cognition and language. The qualifier severe was also shown in the categories of Activities and Participation, Communication, Interpersonal Interactions, and Relationships.

Table 10.1. The ICF-CY checklist

Functioning and Disability		Codes	Qualifiers
Body functions	Mental functions	b110, b114, b122, b134, b140, b152, b167	Severe
		b147, b156	Moderate
	Sensory functions	b210, b230, b235	Moderate
		b260, b265	Mild
	Voice functions	b310	Severe
	Immunological functions	b435, b439	Moderate
	Respiratory functions	b440	Mild
	Metabolic functions	b559	Mild
	Neuromusculoskeletal and movement-related functions	b710, b715, b729, b765	Mild

Table 10.1. Continued

Body structures	Structures of the nervous system	s110	Mild
		s150	Moderate
	Eye, ear, and related structures	s250	Mild
	Structures involved in voice and speech	s399	Severe
	Structures immunological and respiratory	s499	Severe
Activities and participation	Learning and applying knowledge	d110, d115, d130, d131, d133, d160	Severe
	General tasks and demands	d230, d250	Moderate
	Communication	d310, d315, d330, d331, d335	Severe
	Mobility	d410, d415	Moderate
	Self-care	d530, d550, d560	Moderate
	Interpersonal interactions and relationships	d710	Severe
Contextual Factors		**Codes**	**Qualifiers**
Environmental factors	Products and technology	e110, e115, e125	+Mild facilitator
	Support and relationships	e310, e340, e355	+Moderate facilitator
	Attitudes	e410, e440, e450	+Substantial facilitator
	Services, systems, and policies	e570, e575, e580, e585	+Substantial facilitator

To assess his global development, we used the Portuguese translation of the Griffiths Mental Development Scales (GMDS-ER; Luiz et al., 2006), in January 2020. We confirmed a global developmental delay with a significant pattern of low results in two subscales – Autonomy and Social/Personal skills and Language – followed by scales related to global and fine motor skills, with best results in scales of realization and perceptive skills, as shown in Table 10.2.

During assessment, Victor's social interactions with the psychologist were difficult, with avoidant eye contact most of the time, but tactile contact was not rejected. His attention was only intermittently maintained.

Table 10.2. Victor: First assessment with Griffiths Mental Development Scales prepandemic lockdown

Raw Results	Subscale A Locomotor	Subscale B Personal-Social	Subscale C Language	Subscale D Eye and Hand Coordination	Subscale E Realization	Subscale F Practical Reasoning	Global
I First year	12	*11*	*11*	**12**	**12**	12	
II Second year	5	*7*	*3*	**8**	**9**	6	
III Third year	0	*0*	*0*	**4**	**6**	2	
IV Fourth year	0	0	*0*	**0**	**0**	0	
Addition row results	17	*18*	*14*	**24**	**27**	20	120/6 = 20
Developmental age	< 24	< 24	< 24	< 24	< 24	< 24	< 24
Percentile	< 1	< 1	< 1	< 1	< 1	< 1	< 1

Note. Subscale scores in italics are lower scores; items in bold are the highest scores.

Intervention Description

Various weekly interventions were planned within the different deficit areas, by a multidisciplinary team with the parents' involvement and that of the preschool staff. Although all different deficit domains were worked on by all parties involved, we particularly focused on, and tailored our intervention to, each health and education specialist's specificity in the interdisciplinary teamwork. These included language intervention by a speech therapist using the Makaton method (Sheehy & Duffy, 2009), supported by pictures and sign language (Lal, 2010; Bednarski, 2016; Ammawat et al., 2019), and a behavior and cognition intervention by a clinical psychologist, using the Floortime method (Hess, 2013). In addition, there was also an intervention in motor skills with a psychomotricity technician and in early childhood education with a special education teacher.

With the lockdown in March 2020, face-to-face interventions were interrupted, and Victor's parents, who were both teleworking, used and added both specific and signs-adapted learning activities to their daily home routines. Guided activities (songs, telling stories, and culinary and diverse sensorial and symbolic play activities) were sent weekly by email and cell phone links by the interdisciplinary team.

Second Assessment

Victor returned to preschool and face-to-face regular interventions only in September, following recommendations considering his immune syndrome. The second developmental assessment took place at that time. The Griffiths III Scales were used (Green et al., 2016). The big achievement was that Victor started to do an intelligible articulation of the names of everyday objects and actions; he made the transition, during this difficult period with all of its constraints, from a preverbal period to an initial level of oral verbalization.

Despite his progress related to language, the assessment still revealed a general development delay, which reinforced the pattern profile previously presented in the first assessment with GMDS-ER, with the two very low subscales (language and social/personal autonomy). During the reassessment, he expressed great interest in symbolic play and drawing tasks. He started an oral conversation and kept eye contact for a longer time.

The quantitative results fell below the 1st percentile for all subscales, so we used the quartile charts levels for qualitative analysis of items grouped by quartile level of difficulty and the associated construct (Jansen et al., 2020). Using the table and graphic below, Victor's profile showed his strong and weak dimensions.

We could visualize (as shown on Table 10.3 and Figure 10.1) and analyze the items achieved or not and correlate these by expectations for each year. In this case, the Subscales C (eye and hand coordination) and A (foundations of learning) showed a significant number of items achieved, with a dominant fine motor coordination and visual perceptual construct. As we expected (Li et al., 2020), Subscale B related to communication and language (receptive and expressive) and Subscale D related to personal care and emotional and social interaction resulted in low scores.

Table 10.3. Victor: Griffiths III assessment postpandemic lockdown

	Subscale A		Subscale B		Subscale C		Subscale D		Subscale E	
	Item number-quartile	Construct	Item number-quartile	Construct	Item number-quartile	Construct	Item number-quartile	Construct	Item number-quartile	Construct
Year 1	All achieved		All achieved		All achieved		All achieved		All achieved	
Year 2	A2.1-Q1	Contained/ container	B2.1-Q1	Communicative intent	C2.1-Q1	Graphomotor	D2.1-Q1	Social interaction	E2.1-Q1	Postural control
	A2.2-Q1	Contained/ container	B2.2-Q2	Listening attention	C2.2-Q1	Visual motor coordination	D2.2-Q1	Social-emotional	E2.2-Q1	Postural control
	A2.4-Q2	Visual perception	B2.3-Q2	Receptive language	C2.3-Q2	Bilateral coordination	D2.3-Q1	Social-emotional	E2.3-Q1	Balance
	A2.5-Q2	Visual perception	B2.4-Q2	Expressive language	C2.4-Q2	Graphomotor	D2.4-Q1	Social interaction	E2.4-Q1	Balance
	A2.6-Q2	Contained/ container	B2.5-Q2	Expressive language	C2.5-Q2	Visual motor coordination	D2.5-Q2	Personal care	E2.5-Q1	Postural control
	A2.8-Q3	Visual perception	B2.6-Q2	Expressive language	C2.6-Q3	Visual motor coordination	D2.6-Q2	Personal care	E2.6- Q2	Gross coordination
	A2.9- Q3	Visual perception	B2.7-Q2	Expressive language	C2.7-Q3	Motor planning coordination	D2.7-Q2	Social-emotional	E2.7-Q2	Gross coordination
	A2.10-Q4	Visual perception	B2.8-Q3	Expressive language	C2.8-Q3	Graphomotor	D2.8-Q2	Self-concept	E2.8-Q2	Gross coordination
	A2.11-Q4	Visual motor-construction	B2.9-Q3	Expressive language	C2.9-Q3	Fine motor coordination	D2.10-Q3	Personal care	E2.9-Q2	Gross coordination
			B2.10-Q3	Expressive language	C2.10-Q4	Fine motor coordination	D2.11-Q3	Self-concept	E2.11-Q3	Gross coordination
			B2.11-Q3	Receptive language	C2.11-Q4	Bilateral coordination	D2.14-Q3	Self-concept	E2.12-Q3	Gross coordination

Table 10.3. Continued

			B2.12-Q3	Expressive language	C2.12-Q4	Graphomotor	D2.15-Q4	Personal care	E2.13-Q3	Gross coordination
			B2.13-Q4	Expressive language	C2.13-Q4	Bilateral coordination			E2.14-Q4	Balance
					C2.14-Q4	Fine motor coordination				
Year 3	A3.1-Q2	Verbal memory	B3.4-Q2	Receptive language	C3.1-Q2	Fine motor coordination	D3.3-Q2	Personal care	E3.2-Q2	Gross visual spatial coordination
	A3.2-Q2	Color association	B3.5-Q2	Expressive language	C3.2-Q2	Bilateral coordination			E3.5-Q3	Balance
	A3.3-Q2	Visual perception			C3.3-Q2	Bilateral coordination				
	A3.4-Q2	Verbal memory			C3.4-Q2	Graphomotor				
	A3.6-Q4	Visual motor-construction			C3.5-Q3	Fine motor coordination				
	A3.10-Q4	Visual memory			C3.6-Q3	Bilateral coordination				
					C3.7-Q4	Bilateral coordination				
Year 4	A4.2-Q2	Visual perception			C4.2-Q2	Fine motor coordination			E4.1-Q1	Power and strength
					C4.4-Q2	Graphomotor				
					C4.6-Q3	Fine motor coordination				

Note. Items achieved with construct in quartile charts: items with lower scores in italic, the highest scores in bold. Q1 = Quartile level 1, achieved by 76–100% of typically developed children by year age; Q2 = Quartile level 2, achieved by 51–75% of typically developed children by year age; Q3 = Quartile level 3, achieved by 26–50% of typically developed children by year age; Q4 = Quartile level 4, achieved by 1–25% of typically developed children by year age.

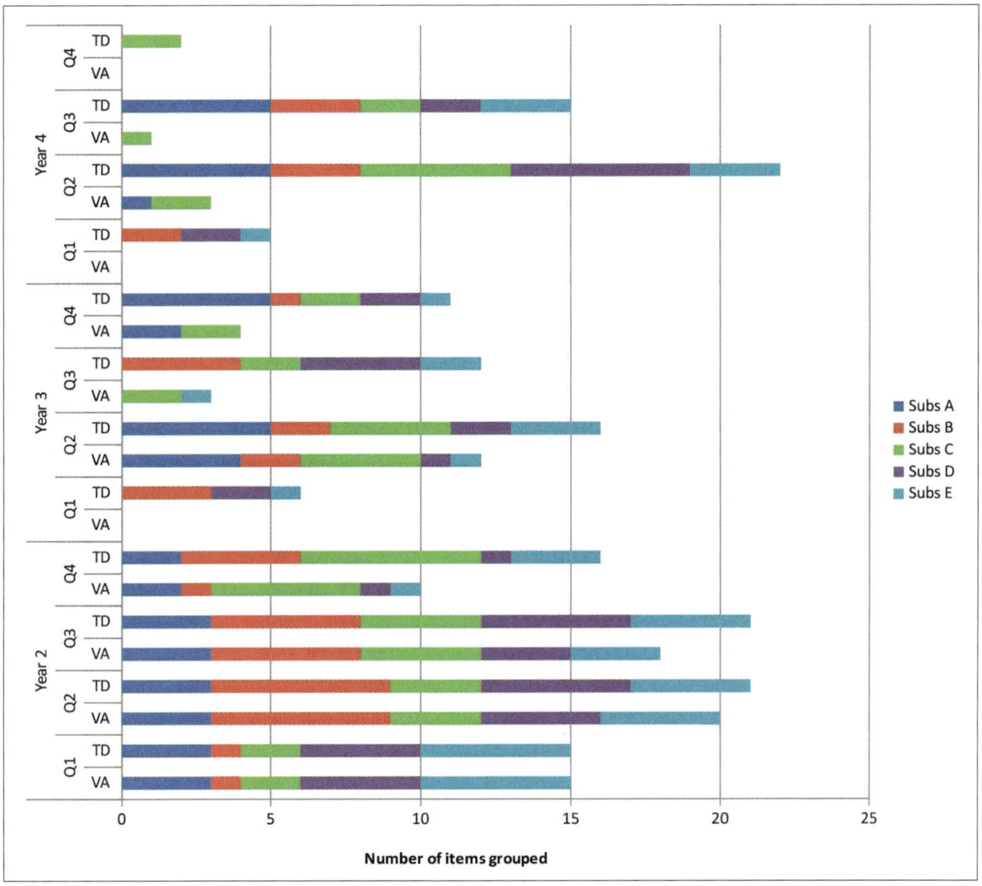

Figure 10.1. Number of items achieved in quartile by year and subscale Griffiths III. Q1 = Quartile level 1; Q2 = Quartile level 2; Q3 = Quartile level 3; Q4 = Quartile level 4. TD = typically developing children achieve; VA = Victor achieved

Check Your Progress

- What was the parents' share of the intervention?
- How did Victor show progress after the intervention?

Connecting the Dots

Autism classification is based on functionality observation. Early assessment is important to recognize and start early intervention (Tarvainen et al., 2020). The Griffiths Scales are an important base to follow up developmental assessment and offer guidelines to intervention in moderate to severe ASD (Li et al., 2020). These are used together with other classifications such as the ICF-CY (Pan et al., 2015) with a holistic intervention perspective, and confirmed by other autism-specific assessments such as CARS (Schopler et al., 2010; El-Ansary et al., 2018).

The indirect and remote intervention with the family by the interdisciplinary team, educational and clinical professionals, despite the constraints during the COVID-19 pandemic (Gruber et al., 2020), was effective, leading us to rethink the old fundamental role of parents (Schopler & Reichler, 1971) and the perspective of an intervention of parent-child interaction in ASD (Scudder et al., 2019).

Additionally, in Victor's case, other comorbid diagnoses were present, and in a behaviorally defined condition that has many different etiologies, it is also necessary to continue the etiologic genetic research (Ramaswami & Geschwind, 2018).

Charting a Plan

In longitudinal studies, plans are charted and reassessed constantly. Victor's intervention plan will continue to be revised as necessary.

Conclusion

Some conclusions we could draw include:

- It is important to use developmental scales with follow ups to the intervention plans.
- Coherence among the profiles was, in this case, demonstrated in both GMDS-ER and Griffiths III.
- In the percentile < 1 quantitative results, quartile analyses promoted a consistent qualitative analysis to intervention plan implementation.
- Developmental scales helped the functional development assessment to clarify neurodevelopment in this complex comorbidity case, when brain imaging tests were normal, and also substantiated the phenotype for genetic research.
- Never give up, even with a necessary social distancing intervention in the face of difficult circumstances like the COVID-19 pandemic; the teamwork with Victor's parents included was a strong factor in his progress.

Discussion Questions

- What do longitudinal studies of development offer that single assessments do not?
- What would have been the expectations of Victor's future developmental progress from his initial assessments?
- Do you think that Victor's parents have recognized their achievement in his developmental progress?

References

Ammawat, W., Attanak, A., Kornpetpanee, S., & Wongupparaj, P. (2019). Pre-schoolers' visual perception and attention networks influencing naming speed: An individual difference perspective. *Heliyon, 5*(10), e02587. https://doi.org/10.1016/j.heliyon.2019.e02587

Baio, J., Wiggins, L., Christensen, D. L., Maenner, M. J., Daniels, J., Warren, Z., & Durkin, M. S. (2018). Prevalence of autism spectrum disorder among children aged 8 years—Autism and Developmental Disabilities Monitoring Network, 11 sites, United States, 2014. *MMWR Surveillance Summaries, 67*(6), 1. https://doi.org/10.15585/mmwr.ss6706a1

Bednarski, M. (2016). The exploring of implementing Makaton in multi-sensory storytelling for children with physical and intellectual disabilities aged between 5 and 10. *World Scientific News, 47*(1), 1–61.

El-Ansary, A., Bjørklund, G., Khemakhem, A. M., Al-Ayadhi, L., Chirumbolo, S., & Bacha, A. B. (2018). Metabolism-associated markers and Childhood Autism Rating Scales (CARS) as a measure of autism severity. *Journal of Molecular Neuroscience, 65*(3), 265–276.

Geschwind, D. H. (2011). Genetics of autism spectrum disorders. *Trends in Cognitive Sciences, 15*(9), 409–416. https://doi.org/10.1016/j.tics.2011.07.003

Green, E., Stroud, L., Bloomfield, S., Cronje, J., Foxcroft, C., Hurter, K., Lane, H., Marais, R., Marx, C., McAlinden, P., O'Connell, R., Paradice, R., & Venter, D. (2016). *The Griffiths scales of childhood development* (3rd ed.). Hogrefe.

Gruber, J., Prinstein, M. J., Clark, L. A., Rottenberg, J., Abramowitz, J. S., Albano, A. M., Aldao, A., Borelli, J., Clark, L. A., Davila, J., Forbes, E. E., Gee, D., Hall, G. N., Hallion, L. S., Hinshaw, S. P., Hofmann, S. G., Hollon, S., Joormann, J., Kazdin, A., & Weinstock, L. M. (2020). Mental health and clinical psychological science in the time of COVID-19: Challenges, opportunities, and a call to action. *American Psychologist, 76*(3), 409. https://doi.org/10.31234/osf.io/desg9

Hess, E. B. (2013). DIR®/Floortime™: Evidence based practice towards the treatment of autism and sensory processing disorder in children and adolescents. *International Journal of Child Health and Human Development, 6*(3), 267–274.

Jansen, J. M., Green, E., Stroud, L. A., & Watson, M. B. (2020). Using the Griffiths III and Quartile Charts in Assessing Autism Spectrum Disorder: A Case Study. *Journal of Education and Learning, 9*(1), 30–40. https://doi.org/10.5539/jel.v9n1p30

Lal, R. (2010). Effect of alternative and augmentative communication on language and social behavior of children with autism. *Educational Research and Reviews, 5*(3), 119–125.

Li, H. H., Wang, C. X., Feng, J. Y., Wang, B., Li, C. L., & Jia, F. Y. (2020). A developmental profile of children with autism spectrum disorder in China using the Griffiths Mental Development Scales. *Frontiers in Psychology, 11,* 3105. https://doi.org/10.3389/fpsyg.2020.570923

Luiz, D., Barnard, A., Knoesen, N., Kotras, N., Horrocks, S., McAlinden, P. & O'Connell, R. (2006). *Griffiths Mental Development Scales-Extended Revised. Two to eight years. Administration manual.* Hogrefe.

Pan, Y. L., Hwang, A. W., Simeonsson, R. J., Lu, L., & Liao, H. F. (2015). ICF-CY code set for infants with early delay and disabilities (EDD Code Set) for interdisciplinary assessment: a global experts survey. *Disability and rehabilitation, 37*(12), 1044–1054. https://doi.org/10.3109/09638288.2014.952454

Ramaswami, G., & Geschwind, D. H. (2018). Genetics of autism spectrum disorder. In D. H. Geschwind, H. L. Paulson, & C. Klein (Eds.), *Handbook of clinical neurology* (Vol. 147, pp. 321–329). Elsevier. https://doi.org/10.1016/B978-0-444-63233-3.00021-X

Rosenberg, R. E., Law, J. K., Yenokyan, G., McGready, J., Kaufmann, W. E., & Law, P. A. (2009). Characteristics and concordance of autism spectrum disorders among 277 twin pairs. *Archives of Pediatrics & Adolescent Medicine, 163*(10), 907–914. https://doi.org/10.1001/archpediatrics.2009.98

Sheehy, K., & Duffy, H. (2009). Attitudes to Makaton in the ages on integration and inclusion. *International Journal of Special Education, 24*(2), 91–102.

Schopler, E., & Reichler, R. J. (1971). Parents as cotherapists in the treatment of psychotic children. *Journal of Autism and Childhood Schizophrenia, 1,* 87–102. https://doi.org/10.1007/BF01537746

Schopler, E., Van Bourgondien, M. E., & Wellman, G. J. (2010). *Childhood autism rating scale (CARS-2)* (2nd ed.). Western Psychological Services.

Scudder, A., Wong, C., Ober, N., Hoffman, M., Toscolani, J., & Handen, B. L. (2019). Parent–child interaction therapy (PCIT) in young children with autism spectrum disorder. *Child & Family Behavior Therapy, 41*(4), 201–220. https://doi.org/10.1080/07317107.2019.1659542

Tarvainen, S., Stolt, S., & Launonen, K. (2020). Oral language comprehension interventions in 1–8-year-old children with language disorders or difficulties: A systematic scoping review. *Autism & Developmental Language Impairments, 5*, 2396941520946999. https://doi.org/10.1177/2396941520946999

World Health Organization. (2013). *How to use the ICF. A practical manual for using the international classification of functioning, disability and health (ICF).*

Zone 3

Zone 3: Children With Symptoms of General Developmental Delay	
Chapter 11	Johan: A Swedish Boy Who Fits the ESSENCE Description
Chapter 12	Sam: Neurodevelopmental Concerns in a Preterm Infant

Chapter 11

Johan: A Swedish Boy Who Fits the ESSENCE Description

Gunilla Carlsson Kendall

The Context

The assessment was carried out at a neuropsychiatric clinic in Stockholm, Sweden, which receives children and adults referred for neuropsychiatric conditions such as attention deficit/hyperactivity disorder (ADHD) and autism. I am a child psychologist, focusing on neuropsychology both from a clinical view but also in the context of informing and educating teachers about children with different cognitive conditions and its impact on learning.

At the time of assessment, Johan was 4 years 7 months old. He was described in the referral as generally delayed in his development, hyperactive, with poor motor coordination, and social and communication problems. The questions raised in the referral were: Autism? ADHD? General developmental delay? Developmental coordination disorder?

- Johan was to transfer from nursery school to preschool in the autumn. In Sweden we have a special curriculum for children with intellectual disability (ID) that might have been applicable for Johan.
- There were concerns about Johan's weak interest in social interaction and poor communication skills, and if he met the criteria for autism, he could be referred to a special unit for more systematic training and support for the parents.
- And finally, if his hyperactivity was due to ADHD, he might have benefited from medical treatment.

Children who do not meet the criteria for ID are generally placed in inclusive environments in local schools. Special schools and special groups exist, but the general idea is that children should be placed in ordinary classes within their age group and receive help with difficulties within the classroom context if possible. For a child with Johan's combination of problems, it was hard to see how he could manage a school setting without adaptations and more support than usual, so guidance before the placement in schools was an important issue.

Check Your Progress

- Why was Johan referred for assessment?

The Child

Johan was the oldest of two children in a family that lived in a suburb of Stockholm. Johan had been generally delayed in his development from the start and was assessed by a speech therapist when he was 3 years old. The speech therapist described his difficulties as a mixed expressive-receptive language disorder, potentially also with oral-motor difficulties. The nursery school and the parents were given advice and information on how to stimulate Johan's speech development. His pronunciation remained difficult for strangers to understand. At the nursery school, hand signs and pictures were used to support and clarify communication. Johan sometimes seemed to benefit from hand gestures, but he did not actively use them himself to communicate what he wanted. He did not crawl, instead sliding on his bottom, and started walking at 18 months.

When he was younger, Johan would often fall and hurt himself, and he still struggled to walk on uneven surfaces without wobbling and falling over. He had low muscle tone, walked on his toes, and often had his mouth somewhat open and might drool. Johan struggled to eat with cutlery, still preferring to eat with his fingers. He was not yet properly toilet trained and wore diapers. He was very active, and it was hard to make him slow down, stop, and listen.

Staff at the nursery school quickly drew attention to his delayed development. He stayed somewhat longer with the younger group at the nursery school but was later moved to the group of older children, primarily due to problems that arose as a result of his high level of activity around the younger children. In that group, it was clear that Johan's abilities were not in line with other children of his age. He had a dedicated minder at the nursery school, and seldom followed regular activities. His parents as well as the staff at the nursery school thought that Johan had made progress over the last 6 months, perceiving that he was more able to take an interest in a few activities for a somewhat longer time, that he had started to communicate more often in two-word sentences, and that he was showing a greater interest in other children than previously.

Check Your Progress

- What are Johan's main difficulties?

The Condition

There is great overlap between different neurodevelopmental and neuropsychiatric conditions and also variation in the presentation of problems, especially in small children. In the last few years, Christopher Gillberg (2014) has suggested an approach to childhood developmental problems that he calls the *early symptomatic syndromes eliciting neurodevelopmental clinical examinations* (ESSENCE). The concept includes ADHD and other early-onset childhood neurodevelopmental and neuropsychiatric problems for which parents seek advice before a child is 5 or 6 years old. These problems include autism, developmental coordination disorder, tic disorder, speech and language disorders, and neurological disorders such as epilepsy. The symptoms can be in the field of general development, communication and language, social interrelatedness, motor coordination, attention, activity, behavior, mood, and sleep or feeding. Children are often referred to a specialist in the field of their current presentation of the problem and do not have the opportunity to meet an interdisciplinary team that could offer a wider range of interventions.

Gillberg (2014) suggests that an early specification of a problem, such as a diagnosis or autism or ADHD, leads to a risk that symptoms not covered by the diagnosis are overlooked. In Sweden, clinics are often specialized in different problem areas: speech and language, or ADHD, or autism, which means that overlapping problems could be overlooked. Thus, a child with several different problems could fall between the cracks. Johan's main problem was likely to change over time: hyperactivity tends to diminish, he was already starting to show more interest in other people than previously, and his intellectual problems may have become more pronounced when he started school.

Given Johan's presenting problems, it could have been hard to find a clinic that could meet and help him and his family. They would likely need to have contact with multiple clinics for different aspects of Johan's problems. Although a referral was made to the rehabilitation center, the only multiprofessional organization in the Swedish medical system, this was declined because Johan had not received either an ID or an autism diagnosis.

Check Your Progress

- Do Johan's presenting problems suit an ESSENCE approach?

The Consultation

The psychological assessment was carried out on three occasions. For the assessment, Griffiths III and the Autism Diagnostic Observation Schedule (ADOS-2; Gotham et al., 2006) were used. In addition to testing, interviews were carried out with the parents and the staff at the nursery school, as well as an observation at the nursery school. Johan's hyperactivity was evident during the test and during the observation, and the assessment had to be adapted to this. When Johan tired of the test on the second occasion, he ran to the door, turned off the lights, and waved goodbye.

Griffiths III Assessment

Johan's performance varied with different types of exercises. He wanted to play with the materials in his own way, and he did not easily follow instructions. He had a very short attention span and moved around the room. Johan performed some tasks spontaneously. He liked the brick boxes and formboards for Subscale A, and the boxes of toys for Subscale B.

Johan named things spontaneously, and the parent had to step in frequently to help interpret his language. After a couple of tries, he named 18 pictures and identified three verbs on the activity pictures card.

On Subscale C, Johan liked putting together connector blocks and building towers. He used the pen to draw a circle and a cross. The results on Subscale D were partially based on information from the parents. He told me his first name and that he was a boy. Even though his parents thought that Johan had become more interested in other children, he did not really play with them in a mutual way. Most of the results on Subscale E were based on observation, as Johan did not follow instructions.

Basal levels for the different subscales were A, 3.5; B, 2.15; C, 3.4; D, 3.5; and E, 2.14. The summary of the basal levels for the different subscales indicated that Johan struggled more with items on Subscales B and E. See Figures 11.1 and 11.2 for the distribution of items achieved for Year 3 and Year 4.

The results on all subscales (except Subscale C) were at or below development quotient 50, percentile 1, and stanine 1. The results on Subscale C were somewhat higher, with a development quotient of 58. The quartile levels for the items showed that Johan mostly performed on level Q1 and Q2 for Year 3, which meant on a level that 51–100% of children aged 3 years can manage. He also managed a few items on Q2, Year 4, on Subscales A and C. The results needed to be treated with caution as they probably did not reflect Johan's full potential but his level of performance in this context.

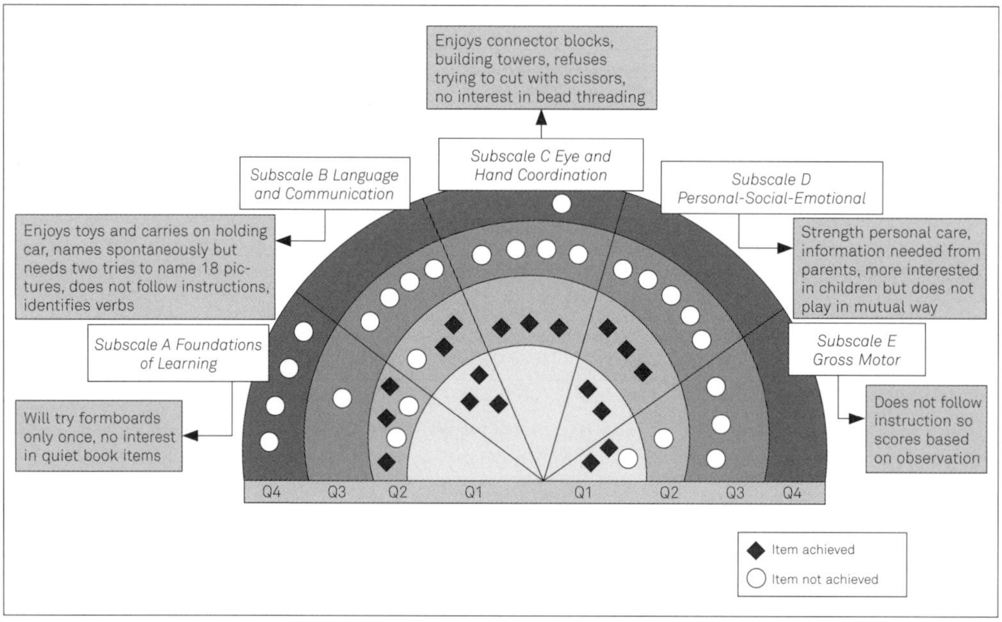

Figure 11.1. Distribution of items achieved or not achieved using the Griffiths III Quartile Chart Year 3. Q1 = Quartile level 1, achieved by 76–100% of typically developed children by year age; Q2 = Quartile level 2, achieved by 51–75% of typically developed children by year age; Q3 = Quartile level 3, achieved by 26–50% of typically developed children by year age; Q4 = Quartile level 4, achieved by 1–25% of typically developed children by year age

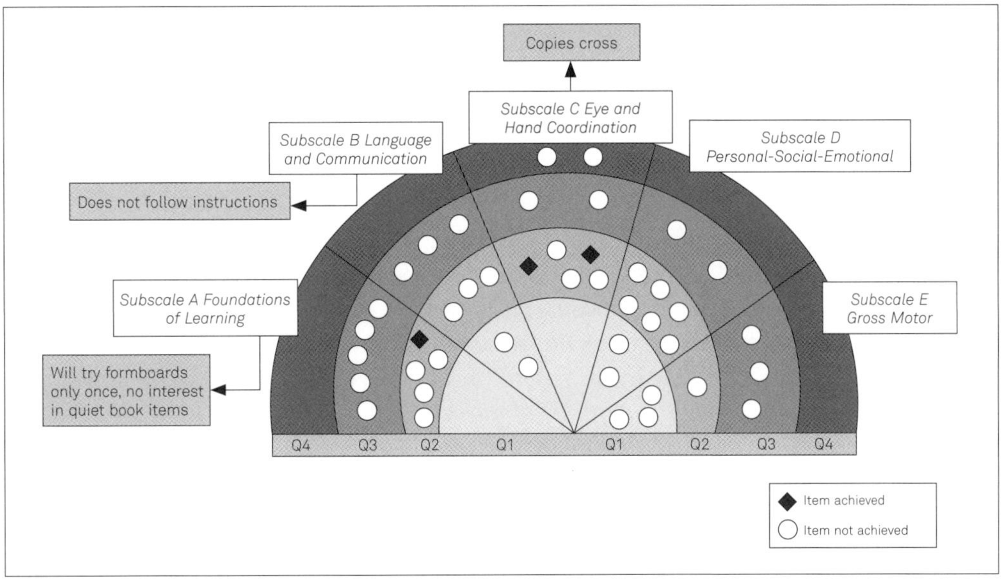

Figure 11.2. Distribution of items achieved or not achieved using the Griffiths III Quartile Chart Year 4. Q1 = Quartile level 1, achieved by 76–100% of typically developed children by year age; Q2 = Quartile level 2, achieved by 51–75% of typically developed children by year age; Q3 = Quartile level 3, achieved by 26–50% of typically developed children by year age; Q4 = Quartile level 4, achieved by 1–25% of typically developed children by year age

Autism Diagnostic Observation Schedule

As Johan made such limited use of language, Module 1 of the ADOS was used. He looked at me, intrigued and entertained, for a short while, as I arranged for a birthday party; he sang along a little and fed the doll once. Johan liked playing with the soap bubbles and the balloons and understood that he needed to work together with me to continue playing. Johan displayed an ability for joint attention, but quickly lost focus. Eye contact was limited, but he could use it occasionally in communication. Johan's results were above the cut-off point for autism, but the results needed to be interpreted with caution as Johan only sporadically took part.

Check Your Progress

- What is Johan's general level of development?
- What aspects of his behavior made assessment more difficult?

Connecting the Dots

Johan's results indicated a considerable and general developmental delay. Even though the results varied to a certain degree between the different subscales, they were comparatively even. Evaluated using the quartile tables, the items that Johan could complete were on a level corresponding to children averaging 3 years of age.

Johan's language and communication skills were limited. However, the parents and the staff at the nursery school reported that he had become more expressive lately and that he seemed able to use and understand visual aids. Autism could not be completely ruled out, but Johan did not exhibit any repetitive or stereotyped movements or actions, and he was not seen as especially inflexible by his parents or by other caregivers (Criteria B in the *Diagnostic and Statistical Manual of Mental Disorders, 5th edition* [DSM-5]; American Psychiatric Association, 2013).

Johan did play in a mutual way with other children, and parents and staff at the nursery school had noticed that he had become more interested in other children lately and could take part in play for brief periods when the other children initiated and organized it. He showed the ability to take turns in activities that he found relevant and showed an understanding of familiar social situations. He interacted with me in a superficial way, but turned to his parents for comfort and help.

Johan's gross motor skills were immature for his age. He was high paced in most of the things that he did, thus contributing to his tendency to fall and hurt himself. His fine motor skills appeared somewhat more developed than his gross motor skills, but when he was eating, Johan tended to make a mess and he sometimes drooled. Johan's ability to slow down and listen was very limited. He was hyperactive and did not often stop and pay attention. At the nursery school, he required considerable attention from staff.

The results might have been seen as representative given Johan's ability to cooperate at this time, but they could not confidently be used to define his greatest potential ability, as his hyperactivity was considerable and affected his cooperation. His general development level appeared to be considerably lower than that of other children of the same age, but it had to be followed up to make sure he really met the criteria for ID. His activity level could not be explained, however, on the basis of his general development level but was so pronounced that it affected his development negatively. He met the criteria for ADHD.

The assessment did not fully support that Johan's restricted social interaction and communication were caused primarily by autism; these could instead have been secondary to his hyperactivity in combination with a general delay in language and general development. Although Johan's results on ADOS reached the cutoff level, his cooperation in the activities was so varied that it affected an accurate interpretation.

In summary, Johan's strengths and needs were that he

- Started to show more social interest,
- Responded to visual aids and start to develop expressive speech,
- Needed help to develop language skills,
- Needed help with toilet training and other basic skills, and
- Needed to have his ADHD considered when designing any kinds of training programs.

Charting a Plan

In Sweden, children start school at 7 years of age, but they start a preparatory year at 6 years old. School is mandatory from 6 to 15 years of age. Johan still needed help to develop basic skills, and there was the possibility of delaying the start of school for 1 year, which might be considered in Johan's case. This decision had to be made in cooperation between the school, the preschool, and the parents. Training can be planned together with psychiatric or habilitation units but is usually provided mostly in the child's ordinary settings such as school, preschool, or at home. Pedagogic support for parents and preschool or school teachers would also have been important to help them understand Johan's developmental level and ADHD. Providing challenges on an appropriate level and helping Johan focus on the things that were happening around him were also topics that needed to be understood by persons in this context.

To promote Johan's communications skills, it is important to design a program that focuses on his short attention span. That training program needs to be built around Johan's interests and create a training environment without too many distractions. The possibility of learning how to interact socially with other children should be facilitated by creating small playgroups in which Johan can participate with support. Medication for his ADHD could be considered to make it possible for him to stop and pay more attention. Johan also needs contact with a speech therapist to clarify the need for training or the use of alternative communication tools. A plan for toilet training should be put in place. After Johan has achieved that, other self-care skills could be addressed.

A follow-up assessment of Johan's development level needs to be conducted in a year to see if he then meets the full criteria for ID. If he does, Johan's schooling would need to be arranged according to the curriculum for children with ID. This would mean that Johan could be placed in a special group in the school or continue to be integrated in an ordinary group but with other goals to reach than the other children, and with more support.

It would also be useful for Johan to get an assessment of, and training advice for, his motor coordination problems. Primary support could be provided by a physiotherapist for Johan's gross motor problems, but also from an occupation therapist to examine if he needs support for fine motor activities, such as eating and writing.

Check Your Progress

- What are the different parts of the plan for Johan?
- Who are the different members of the team that should be asked to see him?

Conclusion

Johan and his parents would benefit from having contact with a center that followed him and his development during his childhood. He has a general delay in his development that might eventually be diagnosed as ID, but problems with communication, social interaction, motor activity, and attention affect his ability to adapt to his ordinary environment.

Johan's broad presentation of problems makes it difficult to differentiate among different conditions – that is, what is affecting what? Does his hyperactivity make it difficult to develop communication and thus to manage social interaction with others? Is his general development delayed so much that it explains his difficulties in language and motor development? Does autism explain the communication problems?

There is a high overlap between autism spectrum disorder (ASD) and other diagnoses. The co-occurance between ASD and at least one other developmental diagnose was 83% in a study by Levy and colleagues (2010). Johan does not reach full criteria for ASD in this examination, but has a presentation of multiple developmental problems that also interacts with each other.

Griffiths III supports a broad assessment and makes it possible to observe how different developmental areas differ from each other while providing a picture of development in a specific field. This was extremely useful with a child like Johan. A combination of the actual results from the assessment and qualitative information makes it possible to use Griffiths III as a tool to plan for intervention. Using Griffiths III at follow-up after another year makes it more possible to eventually decide if the general delay is big enough to fill the criteria for ID. Griffiths III might then also be combined with a traditional intelligence test such as the Wechsler Pre-School and Primary Scale of Intelligence (WPPSI).

An important question to ask is to what extent an early diagnosis of a specific disorder is useful to plan for interventions, or if an early diagnosis that does not fully cover the child's problems could mean that important issues are overlooked. Johan had a speech and language disorder and was diagnosed with ADHD in the current examination. These diagnoses did not, however, fully explain his difficulties. The plan was to do a follow-up after 1 year, when training had been put in place.

In Sweden, institutions that offer help are usually organized on the basis of diagnosis. There are special centers in some places in Sweden for ADHD or for autism, but not everywhere. Parents can find support groups there, but not individualized help. To obtain individualized help for ADHD, you need to turn to a child psychiatric unit, for help to plan schooling there are special teachers and psychologists in schools, and for support for the family there are community-based services. This means that parents with children with problems like Johan have to approach several different services to get help for different aspects of their child's problems. This is often very stressful for parents.

Discussion Questions

- The concept of ESSENCE focuses on early developmental problems that interact and could be symptoms of different neurodevelopmental disorders. Did the concept of ESSENCE cast light on Johan's problems?
- Knowledge of the overlapping nature of neurodevelopmental disorders has been growing over the years. How would services best be organized to meet the needs of a child like Johan?
- What action would you have taken if you had assessed Johan?

References

American Psychiatric Association. (2013). *Diagnostic and statistical manual of mental disorders* (5th ed.).

Gillberg, C. (2014). *ADHD and its many associated problems.* Oxford University Press. https://doi.org/10.1093/med/9780199937905.001.0001

Gotham, K., Risi, S., Pickles, A., & Lord, C. (2006). The Autism Diagnostic Observation Schedule: Revised algorithms for improved diagnostic validity. *Journal of Autism and Developmental Disorders, 37*(4), Article 613. https://doi.org/10.1007/s10803-006-0280-1

Levy, S. E., Giarelli, E., Lee, L.-C., Schieve, L. A., Kirby, R. S., Cunniff, C., Nicholas, J., Reaven, J., & Rice, C. E. (2010). Autism spectrum disorder and co-occurring developmental, psychiatric, and medical conditions among children in multiple populations of the United States. *Journal of Developmental and Behavioral Paediatrics, 31*(4), 267–275. https://doi.org/10.1097/DBP.0b013e3181d5d03b

Chapter 12

Sam: Neurodevelopmental Concerns in a Preterm Infant

Ravisha Srinivasjois, Jason Tan, and Brad Jongeling

The Context

Sam had been a preterm baby who represented, after being lost to follow-up, with parental concern about his development and behavior. He was referred by his GP to a developmental pediatric clinic in Perth, Western Australia, and was seen by one of the authors who was also a neonatologist.

The aim was to address the following objectives:

- Present a preterm child with developmental and behavioral issues and describe how Griffiths III aided in functional and diagnostic assessment.
- Illustrate how Griffiths III can provide qualitative data that aids in diagnostic assessment for behavioral and autism spectrum disorder (ASD) diagnosis.
- Note the importance of long-term developmental monitoring and change over time from early developmental assessments (12 months) to later ones.
- Describe the known developmental risks and complications of premature delivery when associated with brain injury.
- To discuss an appropriate management plan including therapies and further assessments for global developmental delay (GDD).

The Child

Sam was a 42-month-old child who was reviewed with his mother for concerns regarding his speech and language development. Sam, the first of two siblings, had been conceived naturally. The pregnancy was reported to have been uneventful until the mother went into spontaneous labor at 29 weeks of gestation. Sam required invasive ventilation and surfactant administration at birth for respiratory distress syndrome. He suffered bilateral intraventricular hemorrhages (IVH) with Grade 3 severity both right and left. Posthemorrhagic complications of hydrocephalus, or seizures were not evident in the neonatal period. Apart from the IVH, Sam had had an otherwise uneventful neonatal course and was discharged at a corrected age of 40 weeks. MRI of the brain at term-equivalent age showed white matter (WM) loss and changes consistent with previous IVH and subarachnoid hemorrhage.

Given his neonatal morbidities and prematurity, he had been followed up by the early intervention team. Mild delay in achieving gross motor milestones was evident in the first year. Sam started sitting at 9 months and stood without support at 13 months. His mother reported that Sam seemed to catch up with the milestones at the upper limit of normal.

A Griffiths III assessment at 12 months of corrected age had shown gross motor scores on the 9th centile, while the rest of the subscales were in the normal range. His overall development quotient was 92 at that time, on the 29th centile. Sam had been lost to follow-up from early intervention services because the family had moved overseas.

Check Your Progress

- What treatment did Sam receive when he was born?
- Did he have any abnormal signs on his MRI?
- Did he show any delayed development at the age of 12 months?

The Condition

Preterm infants (< 37 weeks of gestation) and particularly those born < 32 weeks of gestation, often referred to as *very preterm infants*, are at high risk of brain injury (Ferriero, 2016; Volpe, 2009). The developing brain of a premature infant is susceptible to injury because of the unique neurovascular anatomy, exposure to infection, inflammation, underdeveloped systems for managing free radicals, and the effects of neonatal interventions (Ferriero, 2016; Hee Chung et al., 2020; Khwaja & Volpe, 2008). Both the gray and white matter may be affected and influenced by various risk factors such as intrauterine growth restriction, infection, hypoxia, and drugs (postnatal steroids) (Ferriero, 2016; Volpe, 2009). WM injuries in very preterm infants range from mild diffuse changes to the most severe form, referred to as *cystic periventricular leukomalacia* (PVL). Cystic PVL affects the brain tissue around the ventricles of the brain and results in scarring with subsequent cystic change.

Apart from WM injury, preterm infants are at risk of IVH, which is classified into various grades based on cranial ultrasound findings and the extent of ventricular involvement (Brouwer et al., 2014). Some severe cases of IVH result in posthemorrhagic hydrocephalus (Khwaja & Volpe, 2008). The higher the grade of injury and the more the prematurity, the higher is the risk of neurodevelopmental complications (Volpe, 2009).

The pattern of brain injury in preterm infants may result in neurodevelopmental complications in infancy and early childhood. The complications may include delays in speech, delays in development of cognitive abilities, and motor delays (Khwaja & Volpe, 2008). In early school age, the observed delays may also include difficulties with initiating and sustaining attention and concentration, with executive function, and learning difficulties.

A recent meta-analysis reported on the association between prematurity and three critical cognitive domains of intelligence, executive functioning and processing speed. The authors included studies of preterm infants with a mean age of follow-up of between 4 years and 17 years. The analysis found that preterm infants performed significantly worse on assessments of intelligence and were 0.82 *SD* below their term counterparts, which corresponds to 12.3 IQ points. Executive function and processing speed were also significantly lower than for their term counterparts by 0.51 and 0.49 *SD*, respectively (Brydges et al., 2018). These findings were seen in younger children (4–10 years) and continued to adolescents (11–17 years).

A population-based cohort study from UK and Ireland followed 315 surviving infants born after fewer than 26 completed weeks of gestation and 160 term-born classroom controls, until early adulthood (Linsell et al., 2018). They found that the preterm cohort had lower mean cognitive scores than their term counterparts at all ages. These studies suggest that the impact of prematurity results in a more permanent deficit rather than a transient early delay (Brydges et al., 2018; Linsell et al., 2018).

Another systematic review highlighted the increased risk of emotional disorders, ASD, developmental delay, and sensory processing delays in preterm infants (Hee Chung et al., 2020). The authors reported that preterm infants had a 2 to 4 times greater risk for ASD diagnosed in early childhood.

Another important complication of preterm birth is cerebral palsy (CP), which is seen in 5–10% of preterm infants born under 28 week of gestation (Hee Chung et al., 2020; Volpe, 2009). An Australian report on outcomes of 22- to 23-week preterm infants found a CP rate of 7%, with moderate to severe cognitive delay in 16% of their cohort (Sharp et al., 2018). This is strongly associated with cystic PVL, chorioamnionitis, and Stages 3 and 4 IVH (Volpe, 2009). Other disorders such as developmental coordination disorder have been reported to have a prevalence rate as high as 37% in preterm infants (Hee Chung et al., 2020). Blindness may be a result of retinopathy of prematurity, which results from the exposure of the retina to oxygen radicals as well as from brain injury (Hartnett & Penn, 2012). Hearing may be influenced by exposure to infections and ototoxic medications such as aminoglycosides. Other outcomes such as sensory sensitivities, signs and symptoms of ASD, attention-deficit/hyperactivity disorder (ADHD) and specific learning difficulties should also be kept in mind. In very preterm infants with comorbidities such as IVH or necrotizing enterocolitis, exposure to high doses of postnatal steroids increases the risk of cognitive delay (Mukerji et al., 2015; Onland et al., 2017; Schulzke et al., 2007).

Check Your Progress

- Was Sam at higher risk of developmental problems because he was born early?
- Do preterm infants perform significantly worse on assessments of intelligence than their term counterparts?
- Is there a higher risk for ASD in preterm infants?

The Consultation

Sam was reviewed after his return from overseas at the age of 42 months. His mother was worried about his development and behavior. She completed an Ages and Stages 3 Questionnaire (ASQ-3) for screening at 42 months of age. Sam scored 2 *SD* below the mean in all the domains of development.

Sam was then assessed using the Griffiths III Scales of Child Development to understand his developmental functioning and behavior. At 42 months, Sam had a limited vocabulary of approximately 10 words. Regarding Subscale B, language and communication, he was unable to put two words together and was unable to speak in sentences. Sam identified and named four objects from six, and identified two body parts. He also had difficulty with comprehension and struggled to follow one- and two-step instructions. He was not able to identify the activity pictures. He was unable to say his name and did not respond to his name being called out.

Sam displayed echolalia and repeated the last word of the instructions. He did not show any interest in pretend play. When a spoon was presented, Sam put it to his mouth. He did not place the doll on the chair and did not feed the doll even when prompted to do so. He had limited nonverbal communication, and eye contact was fleeting. He displayed repetitive behaviors by throwing blocks on the floor repeatedly.

For Subscale A, foundations of learning, Sam was able to complete the three-hole formboard rotated, assemble brick boxes although not by color, but was unable to complete the six-hole formboard. He was able to repeat back one digit but not two digits.

Sam did not show much interest in fine motor activities. He showed an ability to circular scribble and was able to draw a vertical stroke but could not copy a circle or horizontal stroke. He was able to open a screw toy but not reassemble it. He was unable to fix foam puzzle pieces together or undo the big buttons. There was no hand preference. His pencil grip was equal bilaterally but of a primitive palmar grasp type.

For Subscale D, the personal-social-emotional domain, Sam was able to dress himself and identify two body parts. He had difficulty with mirror tasks, was unable to say his name and gender, and was unable to identify facial expressions.

Sam was unable to jump with both feet together off a step. He walked quickly, and there was no waddling gait. The position of his upper limbs was slightly wide. He was unable to squat on the floor on his feet. Sam had coordination difficulties when asked to kick a short tennis ball. At a chronological age of 42 months, Sam achieved the scores shown in Table 12.1.

Clinical examination showed growth at normal centiles. Tightness of Achilles tendon was evident. Deep tendon reflexes were brisk, and Babinski sign was negative. Significant sensory avoidance behavior was also noted. Bilateral talipes was also present.

Check Your Progress

- Did Sam's ASQ scores correlate with his findings on assessment with Griffiths III?
- What abnormal behavior was noted?

Table 12.1. Griffiths III scores for Sam at chronological age of 42 months

Subscale	Raw score	Developmental age (months)	Development quotient	Percentile
Subscale A	29	25	58	1
Subscale B	27	< 22	< 50	< 1
Subscale C	32	24	50–51	< 1
Subscale D	33	24	50	< 1
Subscale E	35	26	52	< 1
General development	31	< 26	< 50	< 1

Connecting the Dots

Sam was significantly delayed in all domains on the Griffiths III assessment, consistent with a diagnosis of GDD. He was particularly delayed in his language domain where he was functioning well below the first centile. Sam had both expressive and receptive language impairment with limited understanding of two-step instructions and limited vocabulary. He showed impairment in his ability to respond to his name, and this together with poor pretend play, poor eye contact, and some repetitive behaviors raised the question of ASD in addition to his GDD.

Symbolic play development as exhibited by pretend play usually emerges between the ages of 18 and 24 months. Sam was functioning closer to a 22- to 26-month level across domains; however, his level of symbolic play and imaginative play seemed below that of his language and other developmental skill areas. His delay in personal-social-emotional aspects of development reflected his challenges with language and with his implicit understanding of his relationship to self and others.

Sam's fine motor skills reflected both his motor challenges and cognitive skill level. He was disinterested in the task, which may reflect both ability and interest. Children who struggle with specific motor or language tasks often avoid tasks they find challenging. Sam's development in this area was delayed – he achieved only half the items that 1–25% of typically developing children achieve in Year 2 and none of the items that 76–100% of typically developing children achieve in Year 3.

Sam's gross motor difficulties were of concern, as delayed gross motor skills are not necessarily associated with GDD. Many children with GDD have age-appropriate gross motor skills or skills in the average to low-average range. Sam had both quantitative and qualitative gross motor issues. The history of significant prematurity with sequelae of bilateral IVH, and physical examination findings of tight Achilles tendon bilaterally was consistent with a diplegic CP. This specific neurological insult was likely to be responsible for his difficulties in motor tasks, at least as they related to gross motor skills, but may have also impacted fine motor areas.

It is conventional to consider corrected age until the first 24 months of life. Hence, correction for prematurity was not considered here. Sam was suffering from GDD, with prematurity and IVH being significant risk factors. Sam also had diplegic type CP secondary to WM changes and IVH.

Although many preterm infants have some signs and symptoms highlighted under ASD, the extent of Sam's symptoms were considered to be disproportionate to his prematurity. Hence, it was decided to formally address the *Diagnostic and Statistical Manual of Mental Disorders*, 5th edition (DSM-5) criteria for ASD, as advised by the Western Australia State regulations. DSM-5 is the main diagnostic system used for addressing mental health diagnosis such as ASD and ADHD. It is similar to ICD-10 coding systems. The regulations referred to here are these that require these criteria to be addressed by three clinicians in order to access ASD services and school support for older children.

Charting a Plan

A family-centered approach with joint decision making and identification of parental goals for their child is an essential part of any plan. This begins by sensitively discussing the results of any assessment and in particular the Griffiths III assessment. In Sam's case, where GDD was apparent, this involved a process of checking with the parents prior to a discussion about whether Sam's behavior and interaction on the day were typical for him.

Prior to any feedback or discussion, we usually ask the following questions: Do the parents believe we saw their child at their best? Did they interact as they would typically at home or in other settings? Did families have any questions or comments about the developmental assessment process or additional information to contribute to the history? Where do the parents feel their child is developmentally, in comparison with peers – at what age level in general, and with regard to particular domains such as language and social skills? This allows the practitioner to consider carefully how to engage the parents in a discussion about GDD or developmental levels, rather than to just jump in.

In Sam's case he had GDD associated with comorbidities including likely ASD and diplegic CP, and he required significant ongoing therapy. After discussion with his parents, Sam was referred for speech therapy, physiotherapy, and occupational therapy. Physiotherapy was arranged to focus on his movement issues including tight Achilles tendons, which would require stretching. A referral to pediatric rehabilitation services was made to consider Botox injections. Speech therapy was arranged to support his language impairments, focusing on his expressive and receptive skills, and use of language in a social context. Occupational therapy was to play a role in supporting fine motor and attention-related skills. These services in Western Australia are supported by referral to National Disability Insurance Scheme early intervention services for team intervention.

In addition, his developmental profile suggested ASD, and he was referred for a team assessment – a combination of pediatric, speech, and psychology assessment to confirm ASD. Following diagnosis, a team approach would be taken using a mix of treatment approaches, including applied behavioral analysis, developmental interventions (DIT/Floortime), naturalistic developmental behavioral interventions (early start Denver model), and other evidenced-based approaches (Whitehouse et al., 2020).

With the interventions, it is possible that Sam might show some developmental catch-up. However, many children with GDD (particularly where significant delay in treatment is present) continue to experience delays and/or disabilities and progress to a cognitive impairment diagnosis (intellectual disability) as confirmed by a psychometric test at preschool age.

Sam would also require ongoing developmental review with a pediatrician as he remains at risk for a diagnosis of attention-related disorders, such as ADHD, and development of a seizure disorder in view of IVH findings on MRI. While it is most likely that his developmental impairments related to his prematurity and brain injury complications, pediatric medical investigations such as chromosomal microarray analysis and other baseline bloods and repeat brain imaging should be considered where possible to rule out other contributory causes of GDD and ASD.

Check Your Progress

- Why is a family-centered approach an essential part of a plan?
- Why was Sam referred to several other health professionals following his assessment?

Conclusion

Sam was an ex-29-week gestation neonate who is now presenting with developmental issues including GDD and ASD behaviors. The Griffiths III test is used here both quantitatively to diagnose the GDD and qualitatively to consider individual domains and interaction – noting both fine motor, language, symbolic and social interaction impairment.

When preparing to assess a preterm infant, it is important to take a comprehensive history of the antenatal and postnatal period. The focus should be on risk factors such as maternal health conditions, resuscitation efforts, infection risk, necrotizing enterocolitis, IVH, any imaging and exposure to postnatal steroids.

Many health services conduct routine neurodevelopmental follow-up of these infants, and it is important to obtain these results to better understand the developmental trajectory of the child. Given that severe sight and hearing loss have been reported in preterm infants, this should be reviewed if they have not previously been assessed as part of the routine follow-up. Physical examination is required to assess for neurological deficits such as cerebral palsy which is increased in preterm infants.

In addition to perinatal risk factors, sociodemographic factors such as parental education and socioeconomic status, and adverse childhood experiences, appear to influence the neurodevelopment of preterm infants. This information will help to identify preterm infants most at risk of adverse neurological sequelae and organize early interventions. There is growing evidence that early intervention may lead to improved cognitive outcomes in this high-risk group (Spittle et al., 2015).

In conclusion, preterm infants are at high risk of brain injury that may lead to adverse neurodevelopmental sequelae affecting motor, speech, attentional, behavioral, and emotional development. A Griffiths III developmental test at 12 months and during later follow-up helps with early identification of neurodevelopmental morbidities and understanding of function, and provides qualitative measures which aid in diagnosis of attention-related disorders and ASD. As seen with Sam, even if the earlier assessments are suggesting age-appropriate development, ongoing follow-up at least to school age should be seriously considered.

Discussion Questions

- What history would you obtain prior to performing a Griffith III assessment in a preterm infant?
- What other physical assessments should be completed in any preterm infant with a history of IVH?
- What nonperinatal factors need to be considered that may influence developmental outcomes of preterm infants?

References

Brouwer, A. J., Groenendaal, F., Benders, M. J., & de Vries, L. S. (2014). Early and late complications of germinal matrix-intraventricular haemorrhage in the preterm infant: what is new? *Neonatology, 106*(4), 296–303. https://doi.org/10.1159/000365127

Brydges, C. R., Landes, J. K., Reid, C. L., Campbell, C., French, N., & Anderson, M. (2018). Cognitive outcomes in children and adolescents born very preterm: A meta-analysis. *Developmental Medicine & Child Neurology, 60*(5), 452–468. https://doi.org/10.1111/dmcn.13685

Ferriero, D. M. (2016). The vulnerable newborn brain: Imaging patterns of acquired perinatal injury. *Neonatology, 109*(4), 345–351. https://doi.org/10.1159/000444896

Hartnett, M. E., & Penn, J. S. (2012). Mechanisms and management of retinopathy of prematurity. *New England Journal of Medicine, 367*(26), 2515–2526. https://doi.org/10.1056/NEJMra1208129

Hee Chung, E., Chou, J., & Brown, K. A. (2020). Neurodevelopmental outcomes of preterm infants: a recent literature review. *Translational Pediatrics, 9*(Suppl 1), S3–S8. https://doi.org/10.21037/tp.2019.09.10

Khwaja, O., & Volpe, J. J. (2008). Pathogenesis of cerebral white matter injury of prematurity. *Archives of Disease om Children, 93*(2), F153–F161. https://doi.org/10.1136/adc.2006.108837

Linsell, L., Johnson, S., Wolke, D., O'Reilly, H., Morris, J. K., Kurinczuk, J. J., & Marlow, N. (2018). Cognitive trajectories from infancy to early adulthood following birth before 26 weeks of gestation: A prospective, population-based cohort study. *Archives of Disease in Children, 103*(4), 363–370. https://doi.org/10.1136/archdischild-2017-313414

Mukerji, A., Shah, V., & Shah, P. S. (2015). Periventricular/intraventricular hemorrhage and neurodevelopmental outcomes: A meta-analysis. *Pediatrics, 136*(6), 1132–1143. https://doi.org/10.1542/peds.2015-0944

Onland, W., De Jaegere, A. P., Offringa, M., & van Kaam, A. (2017). Systemic corticosteroid regimens for prevention of bronchopulmonary dysplasia in preterm infants. *Cochrane Database of Systematic Reviews, 1*(1), Cd010941. https://doi.org/10.1002/14651858.CD010941.pub2

Schulzke, S. M., Deshpande, G. C., & Patole, S. K. (2007). Neurodevelopmental outcomes of very low-birth-weight infants with necrotizing enterocolitis: A systematic review of observational studies. *Archives of Pediatrics and Adolescent Medicine, 161*(6), 583–590. https://doi.org/10.1001/archpedi.161.6.583

Sharp, M., French, N., McMichael, J., & Campbell, C. (2018). Survival and neurodevelopmental outcomes in extremely preterm infants 22–24 weeks of gestation born in Western Australia. *Journal of Paediatrics Child Health, 54*(2), 188–193. https://doi.org/10.1111/jpc.13678

Spittle, A., Orton, J., Anderson, P. J., Boyd, R., & Doyle, L. W. (2015). *Early developmental intervention programmes provided post hospital discharge to prevent motor and cognitive impairment in preterm infants. Cochrane Database of Systematic Reviews* (11), CD005495. https://doi.org/10.1002/14651858.CD005495.pub4

Volpe, J. J. (2009). Brain injury in premature infants: A complex amalgam of destructive and developmental disturbances. *Lancet Neurology, 8*(1), 110–124. https://doi.org/10.1016/S1474-4422(08)70294-1

Whitehouse, A., Varcin, K., Waddington, H., Sulek, R., Bent, C., Ashburner, J., Eapen, V., Goodall, E., Hudry, K., Roberts, J., Silove, N., & Trembath, D. (2020). Interventions for children on the autism spectrum: A synthesis of research evidence. *Autism Cooperative Research Centre*. https://www.autismcrc.com.au/about-us

Zone 4

Zone 4: Children With Syndromes or Genetic Disorders	
Chapter 13	Elena: Assessing a Child With Down Syndrome
Chapter 14	Ben: A Boy with a Mosaic Form of Chromosome 18q21.1 Deletion
Chapter 15	Milly: A Child With Fetal Alcohol Syndrome Disorder
Chapter 16	Ava: A Girl With Phenylketonuria and Typical Development

Chapter 13

Elena: Assessing a Child With Down Syndrome

Silvia Lanfranchi, Chiara Marcolin, Sara Onnivello, and Francesca Pulina

The Context

This chapter has been written by a group of clinicians and researchers working at the Department of Developmental Psychology and Socialization, at the University of Padova, in Italy. Part of this group has worked on the Italian translation and standardization of the Griffiths III scales. In this chapter, the case of Elena, an Italian girl with *Down syndrome* (DS), aged 5 years 9 months, will be presented. She was attending the last year of kindergarten and her parents sought counseling to decide whether she was ready for primary school. To have a broad picture of Elena's skills, her general development was assessed using Griffiths III. The case of Elena will be described to give the reader an example of the use of the Griffiths III scales with children with global developmental delay. Moreover, since DS has an atypical peaks and valley developmental profile, Elena's strengths and difficulties profile will be explored. Finally, her skills will be analyzed to understand whether Elena was ready for primary school.

The Child

Elena was a 5-years-9-months-old girl with DS. She was attending the last year of kindergarten, and her parents sought counseling to decide whether or not she was ready for primary school. To correctly understand this request, it is important for the readers to note that in the Italian formal education system, in accordance with Law 104/1992 and all subsequent legislation and decrees, children with disability are generally enrolled in mainstream school at all educational levels. They are supported by additional teachers specially trained to facilitate their inclusion in the classroom. It is not unusual that parents decide for their child with DS (or more generally for children with global developmental delay) to stay one more year in kindergarten to give them the opportunity to consolidate the foundations of their learning and to decrease the gap with their classmates in primary school.

Elena was the third of three daughters. Her parents were both Italian natives and both had university degrees. The parents reported that Elena had started babbling at 12 months, and she pronounced her first words at about 24 months. The onset of multiword speech, with phrases consisting of two or three words, occurred at about 36–42 months. She started walking at about 20 months. Marked difficulties were reported in the acquisition of sphincter control. Her symbolic play began to be more complex and frequent at about 42 months.

The parents were sensitive to Elena's needs, and they had always been trying to give her stimuli and opportunities for development. Elena had attended sessions for several different types of therapy: speech therapy sessions once a week for 3 years, psychomotor sessions once a week for 4 years, and cognitive training sessions once a week for 1 year.

On our first meeting, Elena appeared cooperative and friendly, she did not appear to be afraid of others, and she liked talking with them. Her language competence seemed better than would be expected in a child with DS.

Check Your Progress

- How old is Elena?
- What is her condition?
- Why did we see the child?

The Condition

DS is a genetic neurodevelopmental disorder, caused by trisomy 21 and affecting about 1 in 700 live births (Parker et al., 2010). The most common features are intellectual disability (or global developmental delay in young children), craniofacial dysmorphisms, and cardiovascular defects (Gardiner et al., 2010), but other physical and medical deficits have also been associated with the syndrome (e.g., hyperflexibility of joints, small ears, hypotonia, obstructive sleep apnea, and hearing impairments; Hickey et al., 2012; Weijerman & de Winter, 2010). Beyond this, a cognitive and behavioral profile, characterized by peaks and valleys, has been described. Communication is characterized by speech and language impairments, with more difficulties in expressive rather than in receptive language (Abbeduto et al., 2007). Visual-spatial skills emerge to be stronger than the verbal ones, but still show strengths and weaknesses: spatial-sequential, short-term memory and visuoconstructive abilities are relatively preserved, while visual and spatial-simultaneous short-term memory, visual-spatial working memory, mental rotation, and closure skills are more impaired (Yang et al., 2014). Some difficulties are evident also in motor functioning: gross motor skills emerge to be better in balance tasks than in run and ball tasks, overall presenting higher scores compared with those for fine motor skills, with particular difficulties in fine motor precision tasks (Memisevic & Macak, 2014; Wuang et al., 2008). Considering the executive function domain, a relative strength is reported in emotional regulation and a weakness in working memory (Loveall et al., 2017). Finally, adaptive skills present their peak in social functioning, their valley in communication, with daily living skills at the intermediate level (e.g., Spiridigliozzi et al., 2019; Will et al., 2018).

Check Your Progress

- What are the main characteristics of Down syndrome?
- What are the main areas of strength?
- What are the main areas of weakness?

The Consultation

To help parents in their decision, the Elena's general development was assessed with the Griffiths III Scales of Child Development. The assessment was made in a quiet room, where the psychologist and the child sat one in front of the other; Elena's mother was present during all of the assessment, sitting in a chair behind her daughter, but not too close to her. From the beginning, Elena interacted positively with the examiner, being enthusiastic about the activities proposed and listening to the psychologist. During the assessment, she was cooperative and engaged in the tasks, showing interest and comprehension of instructions. As a strategy during the tasks, she often verbalized the steps to accomplish the task while doing it. Her attention remained stable throughout all of the assessment; only toward the end, when she was feeling tired, she started to get up from her chair to look for support from her mother. Shifting from one task to another was sometimes difficult, especially when the task or the material were particularly appealing for her. However, as the examiner explained the importance of shifting to another task and motivated her, she accepted the change of activity.

The results are reported here according to the five subscales of Griffiths III, as well as with the accompanying quartile diagram for Year 4, which may provide a further explanation of how scores that fell below the 50th percentile can be interpreted. Griffiths III scores are reported in Table 13.1, where, together with raw and scaled scores, age-equivalent scores are reported. It is important to note that scaled scores show a floor effect (which is quite frequent for individuals with general developmental delay) and are not so informative when they refer to scores at the extremes of the curve. The quartile diagram for Year 4 is shown in Figure 13.1.

Table 13.1. Elena's Griffiths III scores

Subscale	Raw score	Age equivalent in months	Scaled score	Development quotient	Percentile	Stanine
Subscale A	39	37	0	< 20	0	< 1
Subscale B	53	49	3	65	0	< 1
Subscale C	44	37	0	< 20	0	< 1
Subscale D	53	45	2	61	0	< 1
Subscale E	44	38	0	< 20	0	< 1

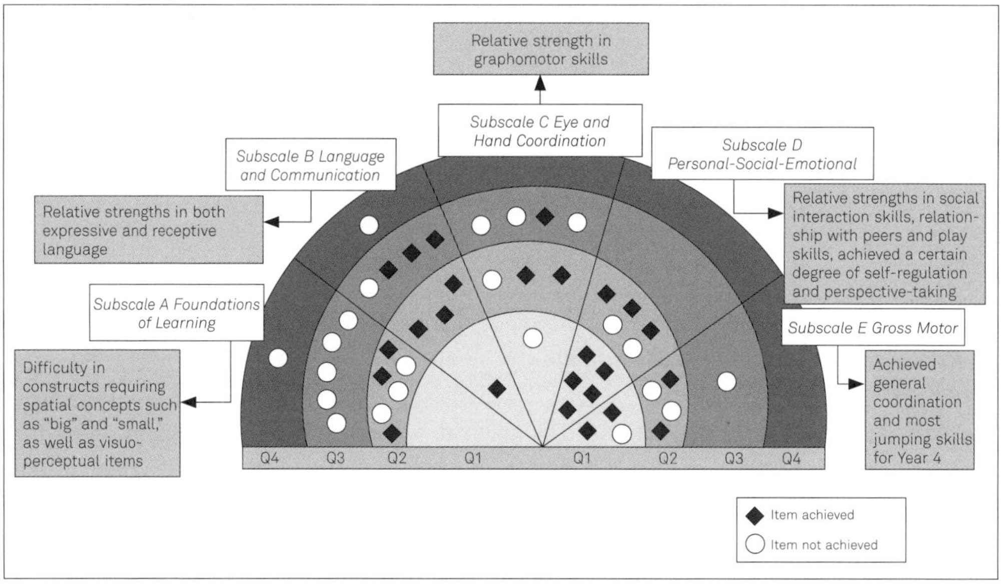

Figure 13.1. Distribution of items achieved or not achieved using the Griffiths III Quartile Chart Year 4. Levels are calculated on Italian normative data. Q1 = Quartile level 1, achieved by 76–100% of typically developed children in Year 4; Q2 = Quartile level 2, achieved by 51–75% of typically developed children in Year 4; Q3 = Quartile level 3, achieved by 26–50% of typically developed children in Year 4; Q4 = Quartile level 4, achieved by 1–25% of typically developed children in Year 4

At the beginning of the session, the psychologist presented the colored brick boxes of the Subscale A, which are useful to understand the global level of abilities of the child and to decide the appropriate starting point. She was able to remove lids and each brick from the three brick boxes and to assemble the brick boxes by color (all 12 pieces); she was not able to build a bridge with the three boxes. This indicated to us that the appropriate starting point was Year 3. Among the Subscale A items, Elena was able to repeat two digits, complete the task of visual learning of the memory house, insert the geometrical figures into the six-hole formboard in 20 seconds, identify 11 target flowers in the object hunt task within the time available (60 seconds), and draw a person with two characteristics. Considering the quartile diagram, it was evident that Elena had difficulties with constructs requiring spatial concepts such as big and small, as well as with visuoperceptual items, which are achieved by 51–75% of typically developing (TD) children in Year 4. Other difficulties were visible for items requiring planning, which are achieved by 26–50% of TD children in Year 4.

During administration of the Subscale B, from a receptive point of view, Elena, identified eight verbs, understood positional words, and followed three two-step instructions out of which two were correct. From an expressive point of view, she named 16 and defined the use of 10 objects from the box of 16 objects, named eight verbs, produced three descriptive phrases from the large picture, took part in a short conversation about something she was interested in. It is interesting to note that some of these skills are expected from children in Year 5 (i.e., taking part in a short conversation) and Year 6 (i.e., producing at least three descriptive phrases and understanding differences). However, Elena still showed difficulties in performing items focusing on verbal reasoning, such as understanding similarities, which are achieved by TD children in Year 4. Finally, she repeated a five-word sentence. Taken together, both her receptive and the expressive language skills seemed to be well developed in Elena.

In Subscale C, Elena was able to draw a vertical line and to copy a horizontal line, a circle and a cross (Stage 1). Furthermore, she demonstrated the ability to create a sausage with playdough, thread 11 beads, hold scissors in her hand, cut a piece of paper with them, and finally, fold a small paper in half. Relative strengths were in graphomotor skills where she completed all of the items for Year 4 (achieved by 51–75% of children for copy-a-circle Stage 1 and by the 25–50% of children for copy-a-cross Stage 1), while the other skills expected in Year 4 were still not achieved, with the exception of folding paper.

Regarding the administration of Subscale D, Elena was able to talk about herself using pronouns such as "I," "me," and "mine"; assume the perspective of the other in the double-sided cards task; and identify five out of six facial expressions. The mother reported that Elena easily separated from her parents and was able to handle frustration by herself. She had more than one playmate with whom she played, even respecting the taking of turns. Concerning autonomies, she was able to dress and undress herself (with the exception of difficult lacing), eat with all cutlery without help and without dirtying, and use the toilet. Therefore, her social interaction skills, relationship with peers, and play skills all emerged as well developed. In addition, good emotional regulation, awareness of self and others, and understanding of others' emotions also emerged as well developed.

Last of all, Subscale E was administered, where Elena was able to walk upstairs (more than four steps) with one foot each step, rise from kneeling without the use of her hands, cross feet and both knees when seated, jump over two 1.5-m (approximately 5-foot) tapes that are 30 cm (approximately 12 inches) apart (first with a single jump, then with a kangaroo jump), throw a short tennis ball into a basket, catch a thrown short tennis ball, and run and kick a short tennis ball through a door made of two bricks. Difficulties were visible in walking along a tape, which is achieved by 76–100% of the TD children at Year 4, walking downstairs with alternating feet, and jumping over two 1.5-m (approximately 5-foot) tapes that are 40 cm (approximately 16 inches) apart, which are mastered by 51–75% of TD children at Year 4, and hopping on one foot, which is acquired by 26–50% of TD children at Year 4. However, it was interesting to note that Elena was able to run and kick a short tennis ball through a door, which is a skill typically achieved at Year 5. Hence, Elena showed a better performance in tasks requiring skills of general body coordination with respect to tasks involving static and dynamic balance.

Check Your Progress

- What are Elena's areas of strength?
- What are her areas of weakness?
- Is her profile typical for a child with DS?
- Why is that, in your opinion?

Connecting the Dots

To sum up, Elena was an Italian child with DS. She was attending the last year of kindergarten, and her parents sought counseling to decide whether or not she was ready for primary school. She was sociable, friendly, and very talkative, an aspect which was favored by a good linguistic development. Indeed, during the assessment she maintained her positivity, being enthusiastic in performing the tasks, following instructions, and keeping her attention on them for most of the time. The assessment with the Griffiths III scales highlighted a peaks and valleys profile, characterized by strong areas in language and communication and personal-social-emotional subscales and weaker points in foundation of learning, eye and hand coordination, and gross motor subscales. This was quite an atypical profile for a child with DS, which reflects the high interindividual variability within this syndrome, variability that can be due to both genetic and environmental factors (e.g., therapies, early intervention, stimuli received from the family, and inclusive school environment).

Charting a Plan

Considering the parents' request, the data collected through child's assessment, observation, and parents' interview suggest that Elena might attend primary school. Specifically, Elena's verbal skills, personal-social-emotional skills, and positive behaviors in response to the examiner's requests, as well as adequate motivation are all features relevant for the passage to primary school. However, her developmental level in the foundations of learning does not seem at that time adequate to support the acquisition of reading, writing, and arithmetic skills. For these reasons, an individualized teaching program together with an appropriate intervention program could help Elena to acquire a developmental level that supports the learning acquisitions of the first year of primary school.

Whichever option is chosen, whether going to primary school or staying one more year in kindergarten, it is important to sustain and enhance Elena's development. By considering her specific profile, Elena should continue with the current therapy sessions, with particular focus on gross and fine motor skills, the latter particularly relevant for several achievements in primary school, such as acquiring the motor patterns for writing.

Therefore, training should be aimed at acquiring higher levels of grasping precision and hand–eye coordination control. Examples of activities are using the playdough and holding and using pencils or crayons of different thicknesses. At the same time, Elena should continue with her cognitive training program, with the goal of improving executive functioning, attention, reasoning, and general learning. The general aim will be to improve Elena's mental age to lay the foundation for the achievements expected in the first years of primary school (e.g., reading, writing, and first steps in math skills). The activities could be aimed at improving reasoning abilities – for example, by using tasks focused on the comprehension of direct and quantitative correspondences (i.e., "If ... then" reasoning), on seriation skills (starting from the ability to discriminate between the greater and the smaller, between two and three elements, and then increasing the number of elements to put in order), or on number acquisition.

Her strength in language skills is very important in supporting learning, as we know that language influences thought. It is noteworthy that Elena's language and communication abilities appear as strengths with respect to her individual profile, but these are not adequate, considering her chronological age. For this reason, even though language emerges as a strength in Elena's developmental profile, it is important to proceed with speech therapy sessions, aimed to sustain and strengthen the abilities already gained and to support the acquisition of more complex and advanced competences. Specifically, speech therapy can be firstly directed toward improving Elena's phonological skills, but also toward developing a more complex and broader vocabulary. Moreover, if at the beginning, the activities are focused on improving phonology and vocabulary acquisition, then it is possible to gradually work on the abilities to compose longer sentences, with attention on morphosyntatic features.

Independently of the specific intervention area, it is important to proceed gradually, respecting the child's developmental stage, and working within the area of proximal development of the child. Finally, Elena's parents could benefit from counseling sessions with a psychologist, who might help them in monitoring Elena's development and skills acquisition and in giving her the appropriate stimuli over the years.

Check Your Progress

- What could be the goals for an individualized intervention for Elena?

Conclusion

The case of Elena shows us how the Griffiths III scales can be useful to assess the development of children with global developmental delays due to genetic syndromes, such as DS. Together with a quantitative approach, which highlights any delays in any developmental areas, a qualitative approach is very useful with these children, showing their profiles of strengths and weaknesses between and within developmental domains. A deep knowledge of a child's skills is very important for planning an individualized intervention, which is particularly important for children with developmental delays and/or atypical development. Moreover, assessment with the Griffiths III scales is particularly useful to assess the profile of skills that are fundamental for school readiness, such as thinking, attention, executive function, language (both receptive and expressive), fine motor skills (fundamental for drawing and writing), and personal-social-emotional skills (fundamental for well-being with classmates). It is important to note that there is not an absolute right or wrong answer on school readiness: Attending kindergarten one more year can have pros and cons – as can going to primary school. It is best to make an individualized decision.

Discussion Questions

- The profile emerging from this case did not reflect the typical profile that the literature on DS describes. The typical profile is characterized by nonverbal abilities being better than verbal ones, while the opposite emerged here. Which variables could have played a role? Do you think that there would have been a different situation without early speech and physical therapies?
- Considering that children with global developmental delay might show a floor effect in one or more subscales, what could be the most informative way to describe their profile?
- If a child with global developmental delay or intellectual disability is assessed with Griffiths III, and if they find it hard to understand the tasks, do you think it would be possible to modify the standard assessment?
- Much information about a child's skills is collected with a Griffiths III scales assessment. How can all this information can be used to plan an individualized intervention for a child with global developmental delay?

References

Abbeduto, L., Warren, S. F., & Conners, F. A. (2007). Language development in Down syndrome: From the prelinguistic period to the acquisition of literacy. *Mental Retardation and Developmental Disabilities Research Reviews, 13*(3), 247–261. https://doi.org/10.1002/mrdd.20158

Gardiner, K., Herault, Y., Lott, I. T., Antonarakis, S. E., Reeves, R. H., & Dierssen, M. (2010). Down syndrome: From understanding the neurobiology to therapy. *Journal of Neuroscience, 30*(45), 14943–14945. https://doi.org/10.1523/JNEUROSCI.3728-10.2010

Hickey, F., Hickey, E., & Summar, K. L. (2012). Medical update for children with Down syndrome for the pediatrician and family practitioner. *Advances in Pediatrics, 59*(1), 137–157. https://doi.org/10.1016/j.yapd.2012.04.006

Loveall, S. J., Conners, F. A., Tungate, A. S., Hahn, L. J., & Osso, T. D. (2017). A cross-sectional analysis of executive function in Down syndrome from 2 to 35 years. *Journal of Intellectual Disability Research, 61*(9), 877–887. https://doi.org/10.1111/jir.12396

Memisevic, H., & Macak, A. (2014). Fine motor skills in children with Down syndrome. *Specijalna Edukacija i Rehabilitacija, 13*(4), 365–377. https://doi.org/10.5937/specedreh13-7465

Parker, S. E., Mai, C. T., Canfield, M. A., Rickard, R., Wang, Y., Meyer, R. E., Anderson, P., Mason, C. A., Collins, J. S., Kirby, R. S., Correa, A., & National Birth Defects Prevention Network (2010). Updated national birth prevalence estimates for selected birth defects in the United States, 2004-2006. *Birth Defects Research. Part A: Clinical and Molecular Teratology, 88*(12), 1008–1016. https://doi.org/10.1002/bdra.20735

Spiridigliozzi, G. A., Goeldner, C., Edgin, J., Hart, S. J., Noeldeke, J., Squassante, L., Visootsak, J., Heller, J. H., Khwaja, O., Kishnani, P. S., & Liogier d'Ardhuy, X. (2019). Adaptive behavior in adolescents and adults with Down syndrome: Results from a 6-month longitudinal study. *American Journal of Medical Genetics Part A, 179*(1), 85–93. https://doi.org/10.1002/ajmg.a.60685

Weijerman, M. E., & de Winter, J. P. (2010). Clinical practice: The care of children with Downsyndrome. *European Journal of Pediatrics, 169*(12), 1445–1452. https://doi.org/10.1007/s00431-010-1253-0

Will, E. A., Caravella, K. E., Hahn, L. J., Fidler, D. J., & Roberts, J. E. (2018). Adaptive behavior in infants and toddlers with Down syndrome and fragile X syndrome. American Journal of Medical Genetics. *Part B: Neuropsychiatric Genetics, 177*(3), 358–368. https://doi.org/10.1002/ajmg.b.32619

Wuang, Y. P., Wang, C. C., Huang, M. H., & Su, C. Y. (2008). Profiles and cognitive predictors of motor functions among early school-age children with mild intellectual disabilities. *Journal of Intellectual Disability Research, 52*(12), 1048–1060. https://doi.org/10.1111/j.1365-2788.2008.01096.x
Yang, Y., Conners, F. A., & Merrill, E. C. (2014). Visuo-spatial ability in individuals with Down syndrome: Is it really a strength? *Research in Developmental Disabilities, 35*(7), 1473–1500. https://doi.org/10.1016/j.ridd.2014.04.002

Chapter 14

Ben: A Boy With a Mosaic Form of Chromosome 18q21.1 Deletion

Hilary Lane

The Context

This chapter outlines a detailed developmental assessment that was carried out by a psychologist who works as part of a multidisciplinary early intervention team in Ireland. The child was diagnosed with a rare chromosomal anomaly antenatally, and he presented with a number of medical and developmental additional needs as a result. A developmental assessment was requested to provide information on his level of overall ability and to ascertain if he presented with specific strengths and needs in his developmental profile to assist with early intervention goals.

The chapter introduces Ben and outlines his rare medical condition. It informs us that Ben's parents received his diagnosis before he was born and details the impact this has had on them. It describes the individual assessment that was carried out in the familiar surroundings of his home environment. His functional performance in each of the subscales of his Griffiths III assessment is described. The information and results are then collated and synthesized. Recommendations are made and an intervention plan is drawn up specific to Ben's identified needs.

The Child

Ben was 2 years 6 months old, the youngest of three children, and lived at home with his parents and older sisters. He had been diagnosed with a chromosome anomaly – mosaicism of chromosome 18q21.1 deletion – a cleft lip and palate, and left-sided weakness, and he also presented with developmental delay.

During the pregnancy, an antenatal ultrasound scan had indicated medical concerns, and Ben's parents were informed their baby had a congenital chromosomal abnormality. He was born by cesarean section at full term and was transferred to the Special Care Baby Unit for medical intervention and follow-up. He was noted to have dysmorphic features and was found to be hypotonic. It was difficult to establish a feeding routine because of this and because of his cleft lip and palate, so Ben remained in the baby unit for a number of weeks before he was discharged home to the care of his parents. Support was provided by the local health visitor, and Ben was seen frequently for regular medical follow-ups in the pediatric outpatient department at the hospital.

At home, Ben was reported to be a "cross baby" who slept little. It was difficult to establish a regular feeding pattern, and he was subsequently diagnosed with significant gastroesophageal reflux. He was constantly in his parent's arms, and he required continual monitoring and attention. At the time of assessment, he was having ongoing difficulties with feeding and constipation. Ben underwent successful lip and palate repair at 18 months of age. He was slow to smile and subsequently had been slow to reach all of his other developmental milestones. He was referred to the local multidisciplinary early intervention team in light of the developmental difficulties associated with his condition.

At 22 months of age, a genetic assessment confirmed Ben's very rare mosaic chromosome deletion. It was considered to be having a significant impact on his overall development.

At the time of assessment, Ben was receiving individual clinic-based physiotherapy and occupational therapy sessions at the local child development clinic. A clinical nurse specialist was calling regularly at the family home to carry out an intervention program and to provide parental support.

Check Your Progress

- When did Ben's family learn of his chromosomal abnormality?
- Why was he referred to the local multidisciplinary early intervention team?

The Condition

Ben had a diagnosis of *mosaicism of chromosome 18q21.1 deletion.* A chromosome 18q deletion is a disorder in which some genetic material is missing, which is known to increase the risk of birth defects, developmental delay, and learning difficulties. For healthy development to occur, chromosomes should contain the right amount of material. People with an 18q deletion have one intact chromosome 18, but the other is missing a smaller or larger piece, and this can affect their learning and physical development. *Mosaicism* is defined as the presence of two or more chromosomally distinct cell lines in one individual.

Mosaicism for a deleted chromosome 18 has repeatedly been found in patients with mostly a full, and occasionally a diminished, clinical picture of the *18q- syndrome.* The 18q- syndrome is one of the more frequent autosomal deletion syndromes. Schinzel (2001) reported that it generally comprises moderate intrauterine growth retardation, facial dysmorphism, moderate mental retardation, and various other anomalies. In an earlier study conducted by Mahr and colleagues (1996), performance in specific neuropsychological functions was consistently in the moderately-to-severely impaired range. Reber and colleagues (1996) found that behavior problems were common, and 6% of patients had autism. There was no relationship between deletion size and any measure of cognition or behavior implications. Vision and hearing are known areas of concern with this condition.

Ben's parents received his chromosomal diagnosis antenatally. Research shows that following a diagnosis of a fetal abnormality, parents can experience a range of emotions such as shock, anger, and grief, as well as adaptation and adjustment. Where termination of the pregnancy is not an option, the process for parents tends to be complex and personalized. It has been reported that some parents struggle to accept the prognosis provided by the medical professionals, doubt advice which does not facilitate hope, and may want to conduct their own research to ensure there are no alternative pathways available to them (Blakeley et al., 2019). A positive experience of the way information is communicated has been described by parents as helpful when faced with uncertainty. In their conclusions, Hammond and colleagues (2020) report that by "ensuring that communication is clear and parents are as prepared as possible, with adequate psychological support provided, we can try to minimize the negative impact of the experience of uncertainty in the prenatal setting" (p. 208).

The National Federation of Voluntary Bodies (2007) developed evidence-based best practice guidelines for informing parents of their child's disability. Though acknowledging that every disclosure is unique, guiding principles include family-centered disclosure; respect for the child and family; sensitive and empathetic communication; appropriate and accurate information; positive, realistic messages and hope; team approach; and planned, focused, and supportive implementation of best practice at all levels.

Check Your Progress

- What is Ben's medical condition?
- Is there a negative impact to receiving knowledge of probable disability before the child is born?
- How can this negative impact be lessened?

The Consultation

Information was gathered from the following sources: parental reports and information, reports from therapists on the early intervention team, clinical observations during assessment, and the use of the Griffiths III.

Clinical Observations

Ben was seen at home in the company of both parents who provided information on his early medical and developmental history and on his abilities as seen at home on a day-to-day basis. Ben presented as an active 2-year-and-6-month-old child. He was observed crawling around the floor independently. His left-sided weakness was noticeable, but it did not appear to restrict his general gross motor movements. He moved about freely, occupying himself with self-selected activities. Ben did not respond when his name was called, but he did appear to hear, and he responded to certain noises. His parents reported a consistent response to some familiar songs and noises. Ben did vocalize from time to time but his vocalizations were without communicative intent.

Ben was also observed in a standing frame, where he was well supported with a tray in front of him, for table-top activities. He remained in the frame for some time once he was engaged with a noisy toy. He became restless after a short time and complained loudly until he was placed back on the floor.

Assessment Results

Ben's general development quotient on the Griffiths III was not calculated, because all of his subscale development quotient scores fell below 50, which was below the floor of the test. His scaled scores were all 0, and his percentile ranks fell at or less than 1, indicating that both his overall level of functioning and his skills, measured by the different subscales, were in the extremely low range for his age group. These results, as shown in Table 14.1 below, indicated the complexity of Ben's needs but did not provide information as to his specific strengths and areas for improvement.

Table 14.1. Ben's Griffiths III subscale scaled scores, development quotients, percentiles, and stanines

Subscale	Scaled score	Development quotient	Percentile	Stanine
Subscale A	0	< 50	1	1
Subscale B	0	< 50	< 1	1
Subscale C	0	< 50	< 1	1
Subscale D	0	< 50	< 1	1
Subscale E	0	< 50	< 1	1

To investigate Ben's abilities and skills and to provide recommendations for further growth, the Griffiths III Quartile Charts (Association for Research in Infant and Child Development [ARICD], 2020) were used. Recommendations from a study titled "Parental experiences of uncertainty following an abnormal fetal anomaly scan: Insights using Han's taxonomy of uncertainty" (Hammond et al., 2020) were also used. Figure 14.1 shows the distribution of the items that Ben successfully achieved, which were all in Year 1 (1- to 12-month level). This quartile chart was therefore used to investigate the specific skills and constructs achieved by Ben.

Subscale A

Examples of the test items Ben successfully completed for foundations of learning were that he reached and took a yellow brick offered to him and passed it from hand to hand. He briefly retained two bricks when encouraged to do so, but he did not combine them or any two objects during testing. He visually tracked a fallen object briefly. He was unable to

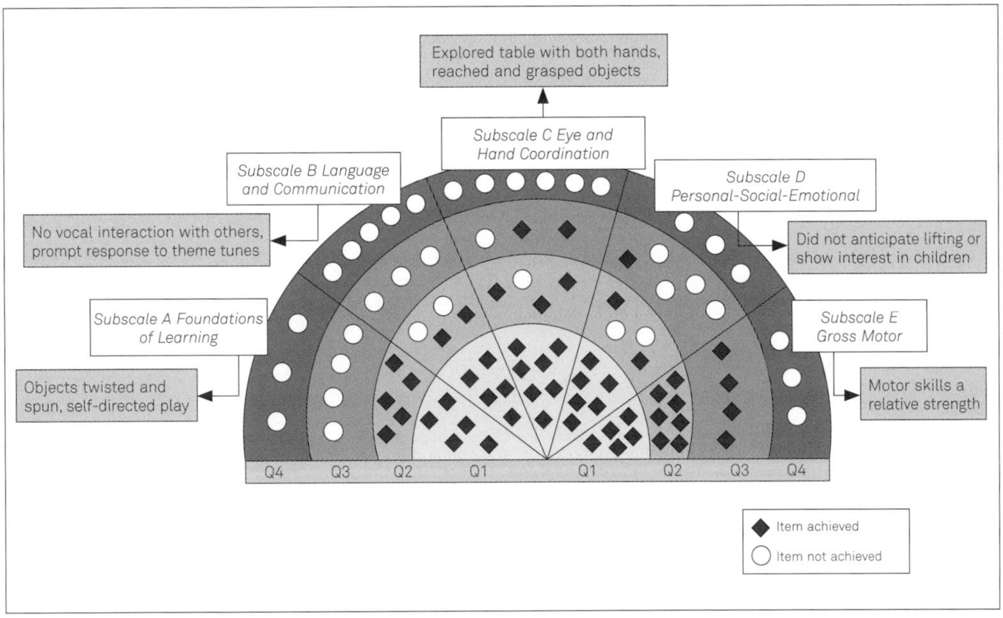

Figure 14.1. Distribution of items achieved or not achieved using the Griffiths III Quartile Chart Year 1. Q1 = Quartile level 1, achieved by 76–100% of typically developed children in Year 1; Q2 = Quartile level 2, achieved by 51–75% of typically developed children in Year 1; Q3 = Quartile level 3, achieved by 26–50% of typically developed children in Year 1; Q4 = Quartile level 4, achieved by 1–25% of typically developed children in Year 1

ring the hand bell or find a hidden toy. Of note was that Ben constantly twisted and spun objects, looking at them intently and showing his excitement by tensing and releasing his hands and jaw.

Subscale B

On the Year 1 quartile chart for language and communication, the test items successfully achieved by Ben fell in the 1st quartile with only two items falling in the 2nd quartile. This indicated that this was Ben's weakest area of development. Though Ben smiled and laughed to himself, he was reported to be a quiet child overall who did not yet interact vocally with others. He made two-syllable reduplicated babble such as "ya ya." He did not show any interest in pictures or books.

Subscale C

On the Year 1 quartile chart for eye and hand coordination, Ben successfully achieved all test items in the 1st and 2nd quartiles. He achieved two items in the 3rd quartile. Test items that Ben successfully completed were that he used both hands and banged them on the table. He watched while activities were carried out on the tray of his stander. He grasped objects then turned and dropped them, showing little interest in them again. He did not yet hold a crayon or point with his index finger.

Subscale D

On the Year 1 quartile chart, Ben's successes in personal-social-emotional skills were more varied. He successfully completed all of the items in the 1st quartile. He did not achieve many items in the 2nd quartile, indicating a particular area of need for intervention. In personal independence areas, Ben drank from a bottle but would not hold it himself. He could hold and bite larger finger foods such as a biscuit or wafer but not small foods such as raisins. He held a spoon briefly but did not bring it to his mouth. Socially, Ben smiled when being sung to by his mother, though he did not engage with her. He looked briefly at himself in the mirror but did not further interact with his image. He did not to show a reaction when his parents came into the room.

Subscale E

Gross motor skills were Ben's strongest area of development. Ben was observed to crawl freely about the house. A left-sided weakness was reported, but he showed no restrictions in his mobility when on all fours on flat surfaces. He pulled himself up to stand and was observed to stand alone briefly when distracted, but he was not yet able to sidestep or move around on his feet using available furniture.

Check Your Progress

- Why was Ben's general development quotient not calculated?
- What was his strongest area of development?

Connecting the Dots

Ben was a 2-year-6-month-old little boy who was born with a rare chromosome anomaly. He had surgical repair of a cleft lip and palate and continued to present with feeding issues and significant reflux. His early development had been significantly delayed in all areas. Owing to the known impact of Ben's diagnosed chromosomal anomaly, a developmental assessment was sought to highlight areas for intervention and to provide information on his level of functioning, so he could access the most appropriate early education facility.

Results on the Griffiths III indicated that Ben was functioning under the 1st percentile across all subscales, meaning significant delay in his overall level of ability. This was in keeping with the research on his condition. He presented with a flat profile of low normative scores so the Griffiths III Quartile Charts were used to provide a profile of Ben's skill strengths, needs, and areas for development to be a target for early intervention.

By plotting the test items successfully completed by Ben, his key strengths and needs were identified as follows:

- Ben's strongest developmental areas were his gross and fine motor skills, which were in advance of his other developmental areas. Ben moved about the floor freely and used both hands but he showed little constructive or directed use as yet.
- The test items achieved by Ben in language and communication fell lowest of the subscales. Ben did not use vocalizations with communicative intent, and he showed little interest in and engagement with others.
- In foundations of learning, Ben demonstrated his skills for learning by being able to hold, transfer, and visually track objects. He had yet to develop ways of thinking by using these skills to learn and further develop play skills. At that time, he tended to occupy himself only with toys of interest – that is, those that spin or make certain musical sounds.
- In the personal-social-emotional subscale, Ben showed mixed abilities with low social interaction ability. Though he liked some sounds, rhymes, and music, these appeared to be enjoyed without reference to where they came from – this is, his parents.
- Along with Ben's overall low level of functioning, he presented with a particular lack of interest in engaging with others, poor communicative intent, and a preference for repetitively spinning objects. The literature on chromosomal 18q- anomaly suggests the possibility of a comorbid diagnosis of autistic spectrum disorder (ASD), and Ben's performance on Griffiths III suggested that further assessment may have been warranted.

Charting a Plan

To maximize Ben's developmental and learning potential, a range of both general and specific recommendations were made based on the synthesis of information gained from all sources in the course of this assessment.

General Recommendations

- Ben would require ongoing specialist intervention in a range of therapeutic areas. These might be accessed in a special preschool to help him progress developmentally.
- Ben was under the care of a consultant pediatrician and would continue to require medical monitoring for the range of complex medical issues associated with his condition.
- Ben's vision and hearing would need to be monitored closely as these are known areas of concern with his underlying condition.
- Though differentiating features of significant intellectual disability and symptoms of ASD remains a difficult process, Ben's development would need to be monitored as he acquired the cognitive ability and language required to assess his social communication and play.
- Ben would have required educational placement in a special school facility which caters for the needs of children with significant and complex needs.

Specific Recommendations

Subscale A

Routine and repetition are very important for learning. Regular daily play sessions where Ben was positioned well in sitting or supported in his stander would be important. Activities included offering him two objects and modeling banging them together, taking objects out of large and small containers, taking rings off a ring stacker, and helping him to finding a (partially) hidden toy.

Subscale B

- Hand an object to Ben, ask for it back with your hand outstretched, and assist him to hand it back to you, giving lots of vocal praise when he does. Give visual cues and repeat the request.
- Though Ben may not have appeared to understand any language yet, persevere with labeling objects and talking about what you are doing, etc. Use simple, repetitive language.
- Look at books together – especially books that have a sensory element such as music or lights to hold Ben's attention.

Subscale C

- Ensure Ben was positioned well before engaging him in fine motor activities. This would be essential to promote good bilateral functioning.
- Use activities with a high sensory element to engage Ben.

Subscale D

- Encourage gradual independence by getting Ben to hold his own bottle and cup. Use hand-over-hand assistance but encourage him to take the weight and tilt the bottle or cup. Guide and support but only give as much help as he needs.
- Similarly guide Ben's hand to bring food to his mouth. Give lots of praise when he succeeds.
- When approaching Ben to pick him up, get his attention and hold out your arms saying, "Up Ben, up." Pause before you pick him up so he learns to anticipate your actions.
- Show Ben his reflection (and yours) in the mirror. Make funny faces, kiss, and coo at your images.

Subscale E

- Developmentally the next gross motor step was to encourage Ben to cruise along the furniture and to walk pushing a weighted toy or chair.

Check Your Progress

- Why were both specific and general recommendations made for the plan?
- How were the specific recommendations formed from the assessment?

Conclusion

This case study report has explored the developmental assessment of a boy whose rare chromosomal disorder was diagnosed antenatally. He presented with additional medical needs such as a cleft lip and palate, a left-sided weakness, and gastroesophageal reflux. His medical and developmental needs impacted Ben's ongoing development indicating significant learning needs. Sensitive communication with Ben's parents was vital at the time of diagnosis prenatally, also following the present developmental assessment, and would be necessary again when discussing his needs in the future.

Discussion Questions

- Ben's assessment indicated that he was functioning below the normative boundaries of the Griffiths III. How important is it to look beyond the normative scores in a standardized test when a child presents with significant delay or disabilities? Why should the clinician be cautious when comparing the development of a child with disabilities with a typically developing child?
- It is very important to analyze all of the data gathered about a child in terms of the Griffiths III test items successfully passed or not. When a child shows a significant global delay in functioning, consider how the clinician can find specific strengths, needs, and developmental areas to target for intervention?
- Ben's particular areas of strength and need may have indicated a comorbid diagnosis of ASD. Consider the challenges of diagnosing ASD in the context of more severe levels of intellectual disability.
- Ben's condition was diagnosed antenatally, and the need for open but sensitive disclosure with the parents was noted. Consider the impact on parents of receiving an antenatal or postnatal diagnosis of their baby's chromosomal abnormality and the possible long-lasting effects of this disclosure on parents and families.

Further Reading

American Psychological Association. (2018). *Guidelines for assessment and intervention with people with disabilities.* https://www.apa.org/pi/disability/resources/assessment-disabilities

Fonseca, A., Nazaré, B., & Canavarro, M. C. (2012). Parental psychological distress and quality of life after a prenatal or postnatal diagnosis of congenital anomaly: A controlled comparison study with parents of healthy infants. *Disability and Health Journal, 5,* 67–74.

National Federation of Voluntary Bodies, Oranmore, Galway, Ireland (2007). *Informing families of their child's disability national best practice guidelines.* http://www.informingfamilies.ie

Pedersen, A. L., Pettygrove, S., Lu, Z., Andrews, J., Meaney, F. J., Kurzius-Spencer, M., Lee, L. C., Durkin, M. S., & Cunniff, C. (2017). DSM criteria that best differentiate intellectual disability from autism spectrum disorder. *Child Psychiatry & Human Development, 48*(4), 537–545.

Pezzuti, L., Nacinovich, R., Oggiano, S., Bomba, M., Ferri, R., La Stella, A., Rossetti, S., & Orsini, A. (2018). Beyond the floor effect on the WISC-IV in individuals with Down syndrome: Are there cognitive strengths and weaknesses? *Journal of Intellectual Disability Research, 62*(7), 593–603.

Shapiro, E. G., Whitley, C. B., & Eisengart, J. B. (2018). Beneath the floor: Re-analysis of neurodevelopmental outcomes in untreated Hurler syndrome. *Orphanet Journal of Rare Diseases, 13,* 1–8.

Small, J., Lewis, A., McCallum, J., & Eastwood, J. (2019). Developmental diagnostic assessment for children suspected to have developmental disabilities: An interdisciplinary model of care. *International Journal of Integrated Care, 19*(4), 277.

Thurm, A., Farmer, C., Salzman, E., Lord, C., & Bishop, S. (2019). State of the field: Differentiating intellectual disability from autism spectrum disorder. *Frontiers in Psychiatry*, 10. https://doi.org/10.3389/fpsyt.2019.00526

Visser, L., Ruiter, S. A. J., van der Meulen, B. F., Ruijssenaars, W. A. J. J. M., & Timmerman, M. E. (2012). A review of standardized developmental assessment instruments for young children and their applicability for children with special needs. *Journal of Cognitive Education and Psychology, 11,* 102–127.

References

Association for Research in Infant and Child Development (ARICD). (2020). *Quartile charts.* https://www.aricd.ac.uk/resources/

Blakeley, C., Smith, D. M., Johnstone, E. D., & Wittkowski, A. (2019). Parental decision-making following a prenatal diagnosis that is lethal, life-limiting, or has long term implications for the future child and family: A meta-synthesis of qualitative literature. *BMC Medical Ethics, 20,* 56 https://doi.org/10.1186/s12910-019-0393-7

Hammond, J., Klapwijk, J. E., Hill, M., Lou, S., Ormond, K. E., Diderich, K. E. M., Riedijk, S., & Lewis, C. (2020). Parental experiences of uncertainty following an abnormal fetal anomaly scan: Insights using Han's taxonomy of uncertainty. *Journal of Genetic Counselling, 30*(1), 198–210. https://doi.org/10.1002/jgc4.1311

Mahr, R. N., Moberg, P. J., Overhauser, J., Strathdee, G., Kamholz, J., Loevner, L. A., Campbell, H., Zackai, E. H., Reber, M. E., Mozley, D. P., Brown, L., Turetsky, B. I., & Shapiro, R. M. (1996). Neuropsychiatry of 18q- syndrome. *American Journal of Medical Genetics, 67,* 172–178. https://doi.org/10.1002/(SICI)1096-8628(19960409)67:2<172::AID-AJMG7>3.0.CO;2-U

National Federation of Voluntary Bodies, Oranmore, Galway, Ireland. (2007). *Informing families of their child's disability national best practice guidelines.* http://www.fedvol.ie/_fileupload/File/Informing%20Families%20Guidelines.pdf

Reber, M. E., Mozley, D. P., Brown, L., Turetsky, B. I., & Shapiro, R. M. (1996). Neuropsychiatry of 18q- syndrome. *American Journal of Medical Genetics. Part B: Neuropsychiatric Genetics, 67,* 172–178.

Schinzel, A. (2001). *A catalogue of unbalanced chromosome aberrations in man* (Original work published 1983). De Gruyter. https://doi.org/10.1515/9783112329047

Chapter 15

Milly: A Child With Fetal Alcohol Spectrum Disorder

Amanda Wilkins and Brad Jongeling

The Context

Milly was an Australian Aboriginal girl who was referred at the age of 4 years for assessment of language delay and hyperactivity. Her carer raised concerns about possible *fetal alcohol spectrum disorder* (FASD). She was assessed by a developmental pediatrician at a regional child development center located 370 miles from Perth, Western Australia. The Child Development Centre there is staffed by allied health professionals including speech pathologists, occupational therapists, physiotherapists, and social workers. The developmental pediatrician and child psychologist visit the region every 3 months. The regional hospital provides general pediatric and neonatal inpatient and outpatient care, serving a population of approximately 30,000 people, of which, 8–10% identify as Aboriginal/Torres Strait Islander ethnicity. Collaborative case management occurs between the general pediatric and developmental services.

The purpose of this chapter is to:

- Illustrate the use of the Griffiths III Child Development scales in the assessment of a young child with possible FASD,
- To demonstrate how quantitative assessment of functional abilities in developmental domains is relevant in considering a possible diagnosis of FASD,
- To describe FASD and its associated neurodevelopmental impairments more broadly,
- To discuss appropriate management and early intervention therapies for FASD.

The Child

At the time of assessment, Milly was 49 months old. She had had known prenatal exposures to tobacco, cannabis, and alcohol. Alcohol was consumed at high-risk levels throughout pregnancy (5 days per week). Milly was delivered at 36 weeks gestation by cesarean section for intrauterine growth retardation. Her birth weight was 2,070 g (4 lbs 9 oz; < 10th centile for gestation), length 44 cm (17.3 in.; 10th centile), and head circumference 31 cm (12 in.; < 10th centile). She obtained Apgar scores of 8 and 9 at 1 and 5 minutes, respectively. She was discharged at age 3 weeks from the neonatal nursery into the care of an unrelated carer, by informal family arrangement.

Milly had a past medical history of bilateral developmental hip dysplasia, treated with a brace from 6 weeks to 13 months. She had suffered recurrent otitis media requiring grommets at age 19 months and continued to get recurrent discharging ears about once a month.

In her developmental history, Milly had started walking at 16 months. Her carer commented that she showed delay in using her hands in the first 6 months. She presented to child development services at age 17 months with concerns about speech delay. At that time she was assessed by a speech and language pathologist who found that her expressive language was in the average range (32nd centile), and her receptive language was in the below-average range (13th centile) on the Receptive-Expressive Emergent Language-3 tool, which is an assessment tool based on parent report. On speech pathology review at age 2 years 8 months, she was using two-three word phrases. She demonstrated age-appropriate comprehension and play. She was discharged from speech pathology at that time.

Milly was a very active child. She was described as "into everything." She was quite impulsive and adventurous. She showed a lack of awareness of danger; for example, in climbing and jumping off high places. She also tended to impulsively run off from her carer. She had a short attention span and was not yet able to pay attention at story time. She could not sit still and did not remain seated at mealtimes. Milly was described as very sociable. However, she did not yet understand boundaries with strangers. She could show overfamiliarity such as in hugging and kissing strangers. Milly made friends very quickly but was yet to establish a close friendship with any one child. She attended formal childcare and was booked for kindergarten the next year.

Milly showed oral sensory-seeking behavior and chewed on paper, playdough, and other craft materials. She had achieved bladder continence but still preferred a nappy for her bowels. Milly was able to undress herself except for difficult fastenings and assisted with dressing. She fed herself but was not yet eating a meal neatly.

Check Your Progress

- What were the concerns about Milly's early development?
- Why was her behavior of concern?

The Condition

FASD is a neurodevelopmental disability caused by the toxic effects of alcohol on the developing fetal brain. The term *fetal alcohol syndrome* (FAS) was first described in 1973 in infants born to alcoholic mothers who had prenatal and postnatal growth deficiency, microcephaly, facial dysmorphic features, and global developmental delay (GDD) and intellectual disability (Jones & Smith, 1973).

Understanding of the effects of *prenatal alcohol exposure* (PAE) has broadened to include a spectrum of cognitive effects and birth defects (Mattson et al., 2019). The severity and type of effects are related to the quantity, frequency, and timing of alcohol consumption in pregnancy and maternal factors such as nutrition (Mattson et al., 2019). The World Health

Organization sites a global prevalence of FAS of 2–7/1,000 and of FASD of up to 176/1,000 (Hendricks et al., 2019).

The intellectual capacity of individuals within FASD ranges from severe intellectual disability to the average range (Mattson et al., 2019). The impairments related to PAE are described within 3 main diagnostic domains – neurocognitive, adaptive behavior, and self-regulation (Garrison et al., 2019). However, in the diagnostic guidelines developed in Australia and Canada, these three areas have been expanded to 10 domains of impairment (Bower & Elliott, 2016) – brain structure and neurology (including microcephaly), motor skills, cognition, language, academic achievement, memory, attention, affect regulation, adaptive behavior, and executive functioning.

Young children may show isolated developmental delays or GDD and behavioral disturbances including hyperactivity, impulsivity, and impaired self-regulation (Garrison et al., 2019; Subramoney et al., 2018). In applying Griffiths III, the practitioner can assess three developmental domains affected in FASD – language and communication, motor skills (eye and hand coordination and gross motor), and personal-social-emotional behaviors (proxy measure of adaptive behavior). The definition of GDD using Griffiths III satisfies the Australian FASD diagnostic criteria for significant impairment in three or more domains (Bower et al., 2017).

The majority of studies of toddlers (24–47 months) have shown poorer cognitive scores in the PAE group compared with controls (Subramoney et al., 2018). However, in a systematic review of studies of infants aged 3 months to 2 years, Garrison and colleagues (2019) found that only 54% of studies showed lower cognitive performance following PAE. In Sweden, Larsson and colleagues (1985) found that at 20 months, toddlers in the highest PAE group had lower scores compared with lower-PAE groups on Griffiths MDS, in the domains of performance, eye and hand coordination, and personal and social development (Larsson et al., 1985).

Study results of the effects of PAE on general development in 4–5 year olds have been varied; however, there is evidence of a dose–response relationship, with higher levels of exposure associated with lower IQ scores (Subramoney et al., 2018). Deficits in executive functioning and attention can also be demonstrated in this age group. Specific deficits in executive functioning include lack of inhibition, poorer cognitive flexibility, and poorer sustained attention (Subramoney et al., 2018).

The language impairments in children with FASD encompass expressive delays, comprehension difficulties, and difficulties with social communication (Hendricks et al., 2019). Longitudinal studies have demonstrated significant negative effects on language development in the first 3 years of life for children with moderate to heavy PAE, independent of sociodemographic and environmental factors (Hendricks et al., 2019). However, the home environment was shown to modify the effect in older children (Hendricks et al., 2019).

A meta-analysis of gross motor deficits in children prenatally exposed to alcohol, reported a significant association between moderate to heavy PAE or diagnosis of FASD and gross motor impairment (Lucas et al., 2014). Gross motor impairments were observed in balance, coordination, and ball skills (Lucas et al., 2014).

Finally, PAE causes congenital eye defects and is associated with strabismus and low visual acuity (Wozniak et al., 2019). Both conductive and sensorineural hearing loss and atypical auditory processing have been reported in association with FASD (Wozniak et al., 2019).

Our case study as presented here suffered from recurrent suppurative otitis media, which is prevalent in the Australian Aboriginal pediatric population and contributes significantly to their burden of disability (DiGiacomo et al., 2013).

Check Your Progress

- What is the range of impairments seen in FASD?
- Are there any major domains of development unaffected by FASD?

The Consultation

Milly had an actual age of 49 months 9 days and was assessed using Griffiths III norm tables for 48–50 months. The assessment was lengthy, taking 2 hrs in total (with a food break), and despite this, Milly managed to stay on task. She was delightfully social and seemed to have a good relationship with her foster mother. Griffiths III was administered in English, as Milly had been exposed to English from the neonatal period. In children of Australian Aboriginal ethnicity, it is important to consider their cultural and linguistic background before test administration. Tables 15.1 and 15.2 show Milly's scores on Griffiths III.

Interpretation of scores in Milly's profile demonstrated a developmental language delay, functioning at a 31-month level and below the 1st centile. In the language subscale, Milly was able to complete all tasks at a 2-year-old level but struggled with some of the tasks at a 3-year-old level. Milly was able to complete some of the expressive language tasks, such as naming six objects in the large picture and 18 of the picture vocabulary; and defining four objects by use. However, she had difficulty with naming objects and activity pictures, talking in sentences of four to five words, or repeating a sentence. She struggled with

Table 15.1. Milly's Griffiths III subscale raw score summary

Year	Subscale A	Subscale B	Subscale C	Subscale D	Subscale E	General development
1	17/17	17/17	20/20	18/18	19/19	91
2	11/11	16/16	15/15	15/15	16/16	73
3	8/10	5/10	7/8	8/10	7/7	35
4	3/10	1/8	3/9	7/10	7/7	21
5	1/9	0/6	0/8	1/6	2/7	4
6	0/6	0/6	0/7	0/6	1/7	1
Total	40	39	45	49	52	225/5 = 45

Table 15.2. Normative scores obtained on the Griffiths III assessment for Milly

Subscale	Raw score	Developmental age (months)	Scaled score	DQ	95% CI of DQ	Percentile
Subscale A	40	38	6	76	76–77	7th
Subscale B	39	31	1	54	53–56	< 1st
Subscale C	45	38	6	76	76–77	7th
Subscale D	49	41	7	82	82	13th
Subscale E	52	49	11	104	102–105	58th
General development	45	38	5	70	69–71	3rd

Note. CI = confidence interval; DQ = development quotient.

comprehension – while able to understand positional words and follow a one-step instruction, she was not able to understand similarities, opposites, or two-step instructions, or define more than four objects by use. Utilizing the Griffiths III base rate table, which gives the degree of significance of the spread of scores, Milly showed significant difference in her Subscale B scaled scores relative to all other subscales, further illustrating the significance of her language impairment.

In Subscale A, her performance was on the 7th centile. This could be attributed to language-loading of certain items in this subscale; however, an alternative interpretation was that this profile also demonstrated developmental impairment. Subscales A and B were both on the 7th centile but above the range of disability. In Subscale A, Milly was able to complete tasks in the third year, including Item A 3.5 comparing bears for size (language dependent task), Item A 3.9 matching task – identical pairs (minimal language task), and Item A 3.10 memory house (1) – visual learning task which requires some language to understand the instructions but is not totally language dependent. However, Milly also had difficulty with tasks that seem somewhat language independent, such as completing Item A 3.7 series (1) and completing Item A 3.8 eleven-hole formboard in 60 seconds. She was able to draw a Stage 1 person (Item A 4.5) and complete Item A 5.1 matching task – by association, while missing tasks in between.

Subscale A, foundations of learning, is a composite of items representing cognitive functions including visual memory, auditory memory, ways of thinking, visual-spatial perception, problem solving, and skills for learning. Milly also presented with symptoms and signs of attention-deficit/hyperactivity disorder (ADHD), which was later confirmed. It is known that children with ADHD may have cognitive weaknesses including low working memory and impulsivity, leading to errors of commission. Items which may be failed due to impulsivity would include Item A 5.4 object hunt (2), other foundations of learning, and eye and hand coordination (Subscale C) tasks requiring accuracy (Item C 4.9 joins dot-to-dot circle and square, C 5.6 trails task (1) and (2) – square and circle, and C 4.8 scissors (2) – cuts out square). Milly's cyc and hand coordination was impacted by her attention skills. She was able to complete a Stage 1 circle (Item C 4.1), but not able to copy a cross Stage 1 (Item C 4.4), complete the button tasks (Items C 2.15 and C 3.8), fold paper (Items C 4.5 and C 4.7), or cut accurately using scissors (Item C 4.8).

Milly had particularly good skills in her gross motor skills subscale (Subscale E) results, with significant difference in scaled scores between her scores in this subscale and her scores in all other subscales. The magnitude of the Milly's base rate scatter (difference between highest and lowest subscale scaled scores equaled 10) indicated that the general development quotient was not sufficient or useful to describe the total set of Milly's abilities, because the spread of scaled scores between the five subscales was too large. Tables 15.3 and 15.4 below provide a description of the analysis of the items across Subscales A and C.

Table 15.3. Item analysis for Subscale A: Foundations of learning

Failed items	Task	Constructs measured
3.7 (Basal item 3.6)	Series (1) – both 1A and 1B correct	Ways of thinking, skills for learning
3.8	Eleven-hole formboard (60 seconds)	Ways of thinking
4.1	Three bears and door	Ways of thinking
4.2	Six-hole formboard (20 seconds)	Ways of thinking
4.3	Object hunt (1) – 11 of 14 flowers (60 seconds)	
4.7	Repeats four digits	Auditory memory
4.8	Train puzzle	Ways of thinking
4.9	Builds castle to model using three brick boxes and lids	Visual constructional memory, ways of thinking, skills for learning
4.10	Eleven-hole formboard (40 seconds)	Ways of thinking
5.2	Numeracy – shop	Skills for learning, ways of thinking
5.3	Directional table	Skills for learning
5.4	Object hunt (2) – 6 of 7 balls	Ways of thinking
5.5	Memory house (2) – button pairs	Visual memory
5.6 (Ceiling item)	Picture arrangement (1)	Ways of thinking

Table 15.4. Item analysis for Subscale C: Eye and hand coordination

Failed items	Task
3.8 (basal item 3.7)	Undo all three buttons
4.3	Do up all three buttons
4.4	Copy a cross
4.7	Fold a 100-cm^2 piece of paper twice
4.8	Scissor (2) – cut out square
4.9	Join dot-to-dot circle and square
5.1	Peg board (1) – puts 12 pegs (60 seconds)
5.2	Sequential finger movement imitation
5.3 Ceiling item	Construction pieces (1) – bolts two pieces together with one bolt

Note. The numbers in parentheses indicate items which appear more than once in the Griffiths III Mental Development Scales. They are different tasks, e.g., object hunt (1) – 11 of 14 flowers in 60 seconds and object hunt (2) – 6 of 7 rows of balls.

Check Your Progress

- Did Milly have a subscale score significantly different to the other subscales?
- Were her attentional skills age appropriate?

Connecting the Dots

Milly showed significant developmental language delay and impairment in eye and hand coordination (Subscale C) and foundations of learning (Subscale A). The lower ability in Subscale A probably reflected underlying cognitive challenges; however, language delay could also have been an explanation. Milly had attention regulation issues and hyperactivity which were noted during the assessment qualitatively and required an extended assessment session. Her profile did not demonstrate GDD.

The diagnosis of FASD includes consideration of physical features. Milly's recorded measurements were weight 16.2 kg (35 lb 11.4 oz; 50–75th centile), height 102.5 cm (3.4 ft; 50–75th centile), and head circumference 46.75 cm (1.5 ft; 2nd centile); palpebral fissures 30 mm in length on manual measurement and mean palpebral fissure length 24.8 mm on photographic analysis (Z score, 0.59; Strömland et al., 1999). She demonstrated upper lip rank 5 and philtrum rank 4 on Lip/philtrum guide 2 (Astley, 2013); and facial photographic analysis confirmed two of three facial features of FAS. Milly had normal palmar creases, no other dysmorphic features, normal heart and respiratory exam. She had dry ear canals and grommets in situ. She had a normal neurological exam.

Milly was deemed at risk of FASD but did not initially meet the criteria for diagnosis as she did not meet the threshold for significant impairment in three neurodevelopmental domains. FASD and ADHD were later confirmed on further assessment at age 4 years 11 months.

In Australia, best practice for FASD diagnosis is detailed in the *Australian Guide to the Diagnosis of Fetal Alcohol Spectrum Disorder (FASD)* (Bower & Elliot, 2016). Assessment involves clinical history (reasons for presentation; individual's strengths and weaknesses; and developmental, family, psychosocial, and medical history), obtaining a history of prenatal alcohol and other exposures (with or without confirmatory evidence), clinical observation, physical examination (growth parameters, head circumference, dysmorphology examination, neurological examination, and hearing and vision tests), use of standardized rating scales, and neurodevelopmental assessment using psychometric assessment tools.

Diagnosis of FASD can be made in an infant or young child under the age of 6 years using the diagnostic algorithm provided in the guide with the following considerations: Assessment of neurodevelopment should be made using age-appropriate standardized assessment tools with consideration of the cultural and linguistic background of the child. It is necessary to confirm that neurodevelopmental skills are severely impaired at clinical cutoff level (< 3rd percentile) in three or more developmental domains. A diagnosis of GDD is considered equivalent to impairment in three or more domains of neurodevelopment (Bower et al., 2017). FASD diagnosis can be made in an infant or young child with microcephaly and all three sentinel facial features whether PAE is confirmed or unknown, even without evidence of severe neurodevelopmental impairment (Bower et al., 2017). This criterion was endorsed in order to enable diagnosis of FAS in newborns and infants, according to internationally accepted criteria for FAS diagnosis.

In the case of Milly, the criteria which were met for FASD diagnosis were:

- Confirmed prenatal alcohol exposure,
- Two of the three sentinel facial features, and
- Significant impairment in at least three neurodevelopmental domains:
  - Microcephaly
  - Language impairment (as documented on Griffiths III)
  - Attention (ADHD diagnosis)

On presentation at age 4 years, indirect measure of adaptive behavior could have been applied since her score on the Griffiths III for personal-social-emotional behavior did not meet the threshold for severe impairment. Further assessment by an occupational therapist employing standardized tools may also have contributed to assessment of the motor domain for the FASD diagnostic process. In children older than 6 years, multidisciplinary assessment is best practice (Bower et al., 2017).

Check Your Progress

- What impairment of skills is necessary to confirm before diagnosis of FASD?

Charting a Plan

The first step in an intervention is to sensitively share the diagnosis of FASD with the family and carers. Parents of a child newly diagnosed with a developmental disability are likely to experience grief, and this is compounded for birth mothers of children with FASD who also experience guilt and shame. In the Australian context, practitioners should be aware that Aboriginal people and communities have been impacted by erosion of culture and intergenerational trauma, and these factors influence alcohol use.

Importantly, the diagnosis of FASD offers the opportunity for primary prevention of alcohol exposure in subsequent pregnancies through health education and increased pregnancy support. Programs such as the Parent-Child Assistance Program (P-CAP) are community-based interventions which commence antenatally and continue mentoring and parent support postdelivery through extended home visiting of at-risk mothers (Ernst et al., 1999; Grant et al., 1996). Other evidence-based interventions for FASD include parent–child interaction therapy and behavioral consultation. An example of the behavioral consultation model is Families Moving Forward which provides structured FASD education to the family and practical support in the home for child behavior (Bertrand, 2009). The key worker also seeks to engage those who care for the child outside the home, such as teachers and health care professionals, in order to create supportive environments.

In our case study, best practice involved a family-centered approach, where the individual intervention plan was informed by the profile of developmental strengths and weaknesses and family goals. In early childhood, FASD interventions target social and emotional development, attachment relationships, and habilitation. Early intervention therapies, specifically speech pathology and occupational therapy were indicated for our case study.

In considering the comorbid diagnosis of ADHD, an occupational therapist also has a role in specific interventions aimed at improving self-regulation. Assessment of the child's sensory processing profile is useful to modify sensory stimulation in the environment. Overstimulation is a frequent contributor to emotional dysregulation. Sensory interventions for hyperactivity include providing movement breaks during class, doing *heavy work* prior to sitting for table activities, use of modified seating (e.g., wobble seat, standing desk), fidget toys, and use of weighted vests or lap cushions.

The ALERT program is a specific intervention aimed at improving self-regulation and has been shown to have efficacy in FASD (Williams & Shellenberger, 1995). This can be delivered individually or in a group setting. It uses pictures or colors to describe emotional and arousal states. However, for our child with language delay, the therapist would have needed to consider whether the concepts could be explained in a way that she would understand. In addition, there are specific social skills interventions for children with FASD (Paley & O'Connor, 2009). In our case study, friendliness was a strength, but Milly required teaching of social boundaries.

Medical management of comorbid psychiatric disorders such as ADHD also forms part of the intervention for FASD. At age 5 years 11 months, Milly commenced methylphenidate IR for management of ADHD, with a positive effect. She also required ongoing medical management of her chronic ear disease. This review of FASD interventions has been limited in scope to those relevant in early childhood and preschool-aged children.

Check Your Progress

- What aspects of Milly's developmental needs are addressed by the plan?

Conclusion

Milly's diagnosis of FASD was based on impairment in three developmental domains – brain structure, language impairment (as documented on Griffiths III), and attention (ADHD diagnosis) – with confirmed prenatal alcohol exposure and two of the three sentinel facial features. This case illustrates how developmental assessment using the Griffiths III can contribute to diagnosis and early intervention for a child with FASD.

Discussion Questions

- What other clinical issues could Milly have presented with (and may still have) that would have been consistent with a FASD diagnosis, and how could these have been assessed? FASD is a neurodevelopmental condition with impairments affecting brain structure and neurology (including microcephaly); motor skills (either fine or gross motor or both); and cognition, language, academic achievement, memory, attention, affect regulation, adaptive behavior, and executive functioning (Bower & Elliot, 2016). Milly may have shown a cognitive impairment on psychometric assessment after age 5 years. Milly could have had a developmental coordination disorder, which a physiotherapy and occupational therapy assessment using a standardized tool such as the Beery VMI might have elucidated. Once she had started attending school, Milly's educational achievement could have been measured using standardized tools such as the Wide Range Achievement Test-5. Memory and executive function measures could have been administered by a neuropsychologist and could have included indirect measures or scales such as the BRIEF (Behavior Rating Inventory of Executive Function). Adaptive behavior could have been measured using tools such as the Vineland Adaptive Behavior Scales and ABAS-3 scales (Adaptive Behavior Assessment System, 3rd edition).
- What are the issues with using a tool such as the Griffiths III in assessing children with indigenous or culturally different backgrounds?
  The Griffiths III scales were norm referenced in the UK and Ireland. There are currently no normed data on Australian Aboriginal children, however the Griffiths III has been shown to be appropriate for use in the assessment of development of urban Aboriginal children (Bennett et al., 2010). Any assessment needs to take cultural differences into account, with cautious interpretation about long-term outcomes. All such children require careful follow-up and repeat assessment with a variety of tools and observation.

References

Astley, S. J. (2013). Validation of the fetal alcohol spectrum disorder (FASD) 4-digit diagnostic code. *Journal of Population Therapeutics and Clinical Pharmacology, 20*(3), e416–467.

Bertrand, J. (2009). Interventions for children with fetal alcohol spectrum disorders (FASDs): Overview of findings for five innovative research projects. *Research in Developmental Disabilities, 30*(5), 986–1006. https://doi.org/10.1016/j.ridd.2009.02.003

Bennett, B., McDonald, J., Knight, J., Comino, E., & Henry, R. (2010). Assessing development of urban Aboriginal infants. *Journal of Paediatrics and Child Health, 46*, 384–391. https://doi.org/10.1111/j.1440-1754.2010.01756.x

Bower, C., & Elliot, E., on behalf of the Steering Group. (2016). *Report to the Australian Government Department of Health: "Australian Guide to the diagnosis of Fetal Alcohol Spectrum Disorder (FASD)."*

Bower, C., Elliott, E. J., Zimmet, M., Doorey, J., Wilkins, A., Russell, V., Shelton, D., Fitzpatrick, J., & Watkins, R. (2017, Oct). Australian guide to the diagnosis of foetal alcohol spectrum disorder: A summary. *Journal of Paediatrics and Child Health, 53*(10), 1021–1023. https://doi.org/10.1111/jpc.13625

DiGiacomo, M., Davidson, P. M., Abbott, P., Delaney, P., Dharmendra, T., McGrath, S. J., Delaney, J., & Vincent, F. (2013). Childhood disability in Aboriginal and Torres Strait Islander peoples: A literature review. *International Journal for Equity in Health, 12*, 7. https://doi.org/10.1186/1475-9276-12-7

Ernst, C. C., Grant, T. M., Streissguth, A. P., & Sampson, P. D. (1999). Intervention with high-risk alcohol- and drug-abusing mothers: II. 3 year findings from the Seattle Model of Paraprofessional Advocacy. *Journal of Community Psychology, 27*, 19–38. https://doi.org/10.1002/(SICI)1520-6629(199901)27:1 <19::AID-JCOP2>3.0.CO;2-K

Garrison, L., Morley, S., Chambers, C. D., & Bakhireva, L. N. (2019). Forty years of assessing neurodevelopmental and behavioral effects of prenatal alcohol exposure in infants: What have we learned? *Alcoholism Clinical & Experimental Research, 43*(8), 1632–1642. https://doi.org/10.1111/acer.14127

Grant, T., Ernst, C., Streissguth, A., Phipps, P., & Gendler, B. (1996b). When case management isn't enough. A model of paraprofessional advocacy for drug- and alcohol-abusing mothers. *Journal of Case Management, 5*(1), 3–11.

Hendricks, G., Malcolm-Smith, S., Adnams, C., Stein, D. J., & Donald, K. A. M. (2019). Effects of prenatal alcohol exposure on language, speech and communication outcomes: a review longitudinal studies. *Acta Neuropsychiatrica, 31*(2), 74–83. https://doi.org/10.1017/neu.2018.28

Jones, K. L., & Smith, D. W. (1973). Recognition of the fetal alcohol syndrome in early infancy. *Lancet, 302*(7836), 999–1001. https://doi.org/10.1016/s0140-6736(73)91092-1

Larsson, G., Bohlin, A. B., & Tunell, R. (1985). Prospective study of children exposed to variable amounts of alcohol in utero. *Arch Dis Child, 60*(4), 316–321. https://doi.org/10.1136/adc.60.4.316

Lucas, B. R., Latimer, J., Pinto, R. Z., Ferreira, M. L., Doney, R., Lau, M., Jones, T., Dries, D., & Elliott, E. J. (2014). Gross motor deficits in children prenatally exposed to alcohol: A meta-analysis. *Pediatrics, 134*(1), e192–e209. https://doi.org/10.1542/peds.2013-3733

Mattson, S. N., Bernes, G. A., & Doyle, L. R. (2019, Jun). Fetal Alcohol Spectrum Disorders: A Review of the Neurobehavioral Deficits Associated With Prenatal Alcohol Exposure. *Alcoholism Clinical & Experimental Research, 43*(6), 1046–1062. https://doi.org/10.1111/acer.14040

Paley, B., & O'Connor, M. J. (2009). Intervention for individuals with fetal alcohol spectrum disorders: Treatment approaches and case management. *Developmental Disabilities Research Revivews, 15*(3), 258–267. https://doi.org/10.1002/ddrr.67

Strömland, K., Chen, Y., Norberg, T., Wennerström, K., & Michael, G. (1999). Reference values of facial features in Scandinavian children measured with a range-camera technique. *Scandinavian Journal of Plastic & Reconstructive Surgergy and Hand Surgergy, 33*(1), 59–65. https://doi.org/10.1080/02844319950159631

Subramoney, S., Eastman, E., Adnams, C., Stein, D. J., & Donald, K. A. (2018). The early developmental outcomes of prenatal alcohol exposure: A review. *Frontiers in Neurology, 9*, 1108. https://doi.org/10.3389/fneur.2018.01108

Williams, M. S., & Shellenberger, S. (1995). *An introduction to "How Does Your Engine Run?.#."® The Alert Program® for self-regulation.* TherapyWorks.

Wozniak, J. R., Riley, E. P., & Charness, M. E. (2019). Clinical presentation, diagnosis, and management of fetal alcohol spectrum disorder. *Lancet Neurology, 18*(8), 760–770. https://doi.org/10.1016/s1474-4422(19)30150-4

Chapter 16

Ava: A Girl With Phenylketonuria and Typical Development

Elizabeth Green

The Context

The Griffiths Scales have a long history of use to check developmental status in children with *phenylketonuria* (PKU; Woolf et al., 1955). I am a psychologist currently living in Massachusetts with a special interest in child development, and a registered user of Griffiths III Scales of Child Development.

Ava was unable to follow up at her usual PKU clinic for her planned assessment as the family were temporarily living in a different part of the country. Her parents looked for a psychologist to conduct a Griffiths Scales assessment, as Ava is due to be starting kindergarten shortly. In order to prevent intellectual disability, Ava had been following a special diet since birth. This involved a very limited intake of protein, together with a nutritional supplement (PKU formula). The assessment had the following objectives:

- To assess whether Ava's development fell within the range of typical development for a girl her age and
- To provide reassurance for her family that Ava's PKU was well controlled by diet.

Check Your Progress

- Why did Ava's parents want a developmental assessment?

The Child

Ava had been followed up since her diagnosis of PKU following screening after birth. Both her parents were carriers of the genetic mutation, but both were unaware of their carrier status before Ava's diagnosis. Her father, an accountant, worked in an office local to their current home, her mother worked as a nurse before Ava's birth. Ava's mother decided not to undertake outside work when Ava was born so that she could supervise her food intake and enable her to lead as full a preschool life as possible. Both Ava's parents were educated to graduate level and had an upper-middle-class income. Her mother was mixed race (Black and White), her father White.

Ava is the first-born child to her parents, who decided to limit their family to one child following her diagnosis. She was born following a normal pregnancy, labor, and delivery at term. Her birth weight was 3,300 g (7 lb 4.5 oz). There had been no developmental concerns, and Ava was confirmed to be developing in a similar way to other children of her age by regular developmental assessments as part of her routine PKU care. Ava attended preschool 3 days a week and a transfer to full-day kindergarten at the local neighborhood school was planned for the fall now that she was 5 years old.

Check Your Progress

- What changes to their lives did Ava's parents make because of her diagnosis?
- What effect do you think these changes had on the child?

The Condition

Typical Development

A formal definition of *typical development* can be given as when a child achieves physical, cognitive, language, and social developmental milestones at the same rate as other children of their age, population, and culture. Periods of plateau in development can be followed by bursts of new skill attainment. Typical development is nonlinear and does not occur at a constant rate, and variability occurs both within one child and across many children, with different children developing different abilities. During infancy, normal development is characterized by great variability in performance, developmental sequences, and relationships. If variability is absent with stereotyped performance, and strong relationships between the various motor functions, reactions, and reflexes, this should arouse the suspicion that there may be a disturbance in development (Touwen, 1993).

These unstable developmental changes make the measurement of young children unique from that for much older children (Bedford et al., 2013). The traditional theoretical interpretations of intraindividual variability in early development were that variability is a result of context changes or that variability is caused by measurement error (van Dijk & van Geert, 2014). A more modern theoretical framework, *dynamic systems theory* (DST), sees variability as an intrinsic property of development (Smith & Thelen, 1993). DST has been applied to the motor domain, to cognitive and language development, and to socioemotional development. For the first few years of life, these domains are interconnected, and the major transitions in development occur in a dynamic interaction between the child, the social environment, and the context. Therefore, any measurement of skills within these developmental domains cannot be accurate to a high degree but must consider many factors including variability of skills across contexts. Motor development, in particular, is both varied and variable (Adolph et al., 2015; Eldred & Darrah, 2010 & Hadders-Algra, 2010). There are also many conditions that can impact on a child's development and hinder the achievement of this goal, such as PKU.

Phenylketonuria

Phenylketonuria (PKU) is a rare inherited disorder which causes an amino acid called *phenylalanine* to build up in the body. In PKU, there is a defect in the gene that normally assists in the creation of the enzyme needed to break down phenylalanine obtained from food. About 1 in 15,000 children with PKU are born in the US each year. New-born screening for PKU is required in all 50 states. If treatment starts in the first 2 or 3 weeks of life, and the diet is strictly followed, a child with PKU may develop normally. Symptoms of PKU may be mild or severe and include delayed development or intellectual disability, hyperactivity, behavioral, emotional and social problems, microcephaly, psychiatric disorders, and neurological problems including seizures. There are no gender differences in risk factor or the severity of PKU. Children with untreated PKU have fair skin and blue eyes, as phenylalanine is unable to transform into the pigment melanin.

Check Your Progress

- How variable is typical development?
- What would alert you to abnormal development even with achievement of normal milestones?
- Why is diet so important in PKU?

The Consultation

Ava arrived for her assessment at our clinic accompanied by her mother. Ava appeared happy to meet me and quickly settled down to following my instructions for the tasks of Griffiths III. On the Griffiths III Scales of Child Development, Ava, with a rounded age of 63 months, scored as shown in Table 16.1.

Table 16.1. Ava's scores for Griffiths III

Subscale	Scaled score	Development quotient	Percentile	Stanine	Developmental age (months)
Subscale A	12	110 Range 108–113	73	7	67
Subscale B	11	103 Range 101–105	57	6	65
Subscale C	10	98 Range 97–99	45	5	61
Subscale D	12	111 Range 108–113	74	7	71
Subscale E	9	93 Range 92–95	33	4	58
General development	10	100 Range 99–101	49	5	63

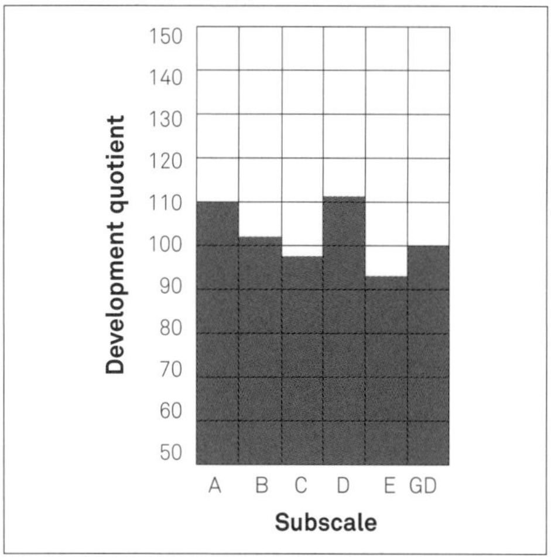

Figure 16.1. Development quotient profile. GD = general development

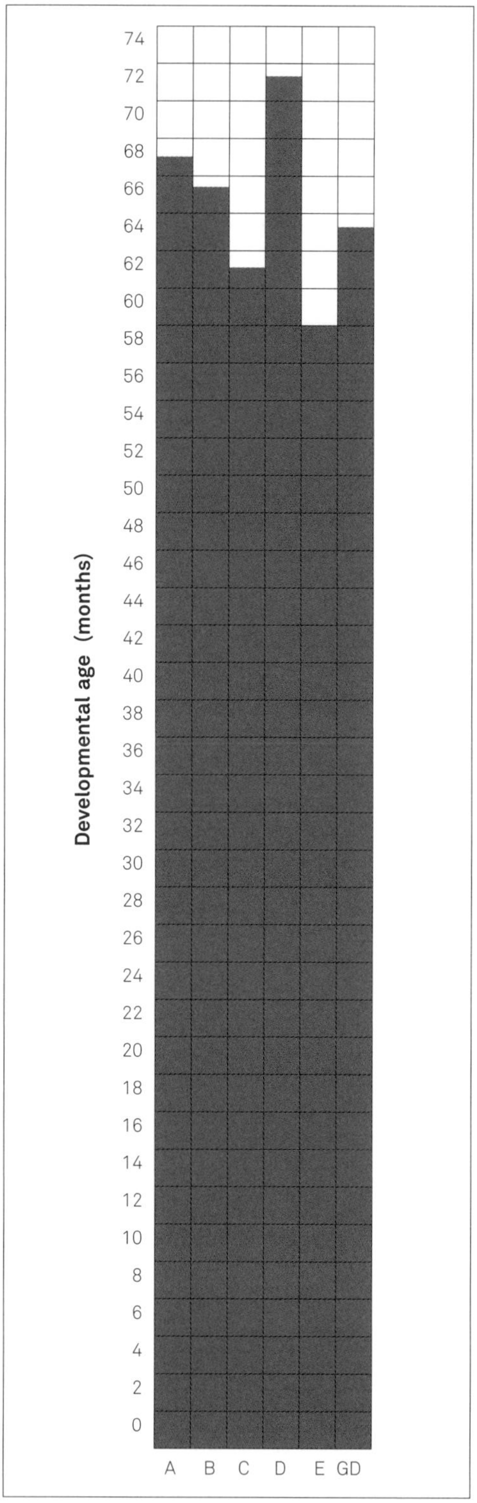

Figure 16.2. Developmental age profile. GD = general development

Base rate analysis confirmed that she did not demonstrate any significant differences between her scores on individual subscales. She did show some relative strengths, but as the interscale scatter of subscale scaled scores was limited to 3, use of the general development quotient (DQ) was appropriate. Figure 16.1 shows her DQ profile, and Figure 16.2 shows her developmental age profile.

Subscale A

Ava was able to complete all of the items in Year 5 except for a memory house – button pairs. Successfully achieved items included patternmaking, object hunt, and spot-the-difference. For Year 6, Ava completed the higher-level picture arrangement item and a memory task. Her drawing of a person is shown in Figure 16.3. She was not able to complete the six-hole formboard within 10 seconds, repeat five digits, or repeat three digits backwards.

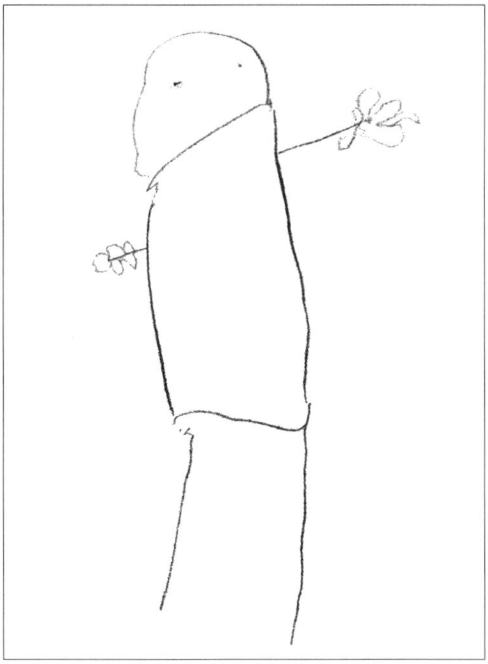

Figure 16.3. Subscale A: Draw a person.

Subscale B

Ava appeared to enjoy the tasks on the subscale language and communication particularly. She was able to repeat a 10-word sentence, understood opposites and similarities, and followed a complex three-part command.

Ava telling a story from the large picture

- *People are driving in a car. The girl is sitting on a chair. The children are playing with a flowery ball. It's good to water your plants so they can grow.*

Understands similarities
- "How are a bee and a butterfly alike/the same?" Ava: "They both got wings to fly with."
- "How are a car and a bus alike/the same?" Ava: "They both have wheel to drive around with."
- "How are a door and a window alike/the same?" Ava: "They both can open."

Word definitions
- Shoe. Ava: "Put it on feet so you can't get hurt on stones."
- Bike. Ava: "You ride on it and it has wheels."
- Horse. Ava: "You ride them as they are big animals."

Subscale C

Ava was able to complete the construction pieces items, peg board and peg items, and laced 80 holes in 60 seconds. However, although she could copy a cross, she was not able to copy a circle with a good shape that was neatly closed or a triangle, or complete the trails items or cut around a complex shape.

Subscale D

Ava's mother reported that Ava could dress and undress, wash her hands and face, use the bathroom without assistance, and eat without making a mess. Ava both named and identified five of the facial expressions – happy, sad, surprised, angry, and cross. She completed all of the moral reasoning and perspective tasks but did not know her address, nor could she talk about herself when asked about her characteristics or personality traits.

Subscale E

Ava was able to complete the balance items, such as hop and kick and standing on one foot for 10 seconds but had more difficulty with visual-spatial tasks such as bouncing and catching the short tennis ball or throwing the short tennis ball up and catching it. Motor sequencing items were age appropriate.

Check Your Progress

- How was it shown that Ava did not have any significant differences in her subscale scores?

Connecting the Dots

Ava had a genetic condition (PKU) which, if left untreated, has been shown to result in severe intellectual disability. She was 5 years 3 months at that time, and was due for a developmental review before her planned start to school later in the year. However, the family were living in Massachusetts, a considerable distance from the PKU service who had planned to review her development. A specialist PKU service has a range of multidisciplinary professionals who have the experience to support both child and family in the management of this lifelong disease. The family did not know how long they were likely to remain in Massachusetts and had not transferred to the local PKU clinic. Starting kindergarten is a time of marked change for any child, so additional support for Ava and her family and her kindergarten staff were likely to be helpful.

Ava's parents had followed the history of the first dietary management of PKU back in the 1950s and were keen to use the modern version of the developmental scales which had confirmed the diet's ability to prevent intellectual deterioration in children.

Transfer to kindergarten would involve explanation of Ava's genetic condition and the importance of her special diet to the staff. She would require an individualized health care plan (known as an IHCP) focusing on Ava's special diet during school and school-related activities.

Assessment using the Griffiths III Scales of Child Development confirmed that Ava's development was typical for a child her age. She did show some variability between subscales, but this was not statistically significant. Her strengths were in the more cognitive tasks of the foundations of learning subscale and also in personal-social-emotional development. Her skills in gross motor visual-spatial tasks were less well developed but still within the typically developing range for her age.

These findings from the assessment were very similar to the comments made by Ava's parents and staff from her preschool, regarding her development.

Box 16.1. Ava's key strengths and needs

- Ava has strengths in the critical aspects of learning which lay the foundation for successful learning and education at school
- Attention and processing skill
- Aspects of executive function such as flexibility, curiosity, and creativity
- Ways of thinking such as reasoning, organising information and planning solutions, concept formation, critical and analytical thought, sequencing, matching, sorting, and finding patterns
- Various types of memory
- Play in terms of engaging real objects in imaginary ways
- Ava demonstrates good independence skills, social interaction with her peer group and emotional development which should aid her entry into more formal education
- Her relatively less good gross motor visual-spatial skills will benefit from the more formal physical games in kindergarten

Charting a Plan

- Ava's parents were encouraged to share this report on Ava's current development with both the staff at her future kindergarten and the PKU service looking after her long-term treatment.
- A local PKU service would be able to help both Ava and her parents with her transfer to kindergarten, so Ava's family were advised to secure this transfer as soon as possible.
- Ava's kindergarten would benefit from literature and specialist input if this was required, from the PKU clinic.
- Ava's parents should contact the school nurse to request that an IHCP was prepared and that there was a joint meeting with them and relevant school staff in preparation for Ava's start there.
- During the summer months before starting school, Ava's less strong gross motor development would benefit from activities such as games involving throwing and catching a ball.
- Ava's family, particularly her mother, may need added support, as some of the dietary responsibilities are passed to third parties in kindergarten.
- Ava herself, though currently developing as other children her age regarding independence, self-help skills, and emotional skills, might benefit from added support, such as from a school counselor as she moves into a different era of her life.

Check Your Progress

- Why should Ava's kindergarten and school have information on PKU?
- What would you expect to see on her IHCP?

Conclusion

Ava has a lifelong disease, which will require her to have a different diet to that of her contemporaries for the rest of her life to prevent damage to her brain from the toxic effects of phenylalanine. Ava's parents had made every effort to ensure that Ava's brain development was not impaired from the genetic disorder which she had inherited from both parents. The assessment using the Griffiths III Scales of Child Development confirmed that her overall development was typical for a child of her age. Her mother had given up her career as a nurse to supervise Ava's extreme dietary needs. Ava's start at kindergarten will be potentially difficult for both her mother and Ava in this respect.

Discussion Questions

- Why do you think Ava's parents may need extra support at this time of transition for Ava?
- Ava's DQ for Subscale A was 110, for Subscale B, it was 111; both had with a range of 108–113. Her DQ for Subscale E was 93, range 92–95. How is the level of significance of this difference tested?
- Visual motor problems such as a difficulty with ball skills could have signified that Ava did have some subtle neurological damage, perhaps from dietary lapses. How would you manage this possibility with Ava's parents?

Further Reading

Carpenter, K., Wittkowski, A., Hare, D. J., Medford, E., Rust, S., Jones, S. A., & Smith, D. M. (2018). Parenting a child with phenylketonuria (PKU): An interpretative phenomenological analysis (IPA) of the experience of parents. *Journal of Genetic Counseling, 27*(5), 1074–1086. https://doi.org/10.1007/s10897-018-0227-7

Chapman, M. (2020, August 13). Tips for parents with children with PKU entering nursery or school. *Phenylketonuria News*. https://phenylketonurianews.com/2020/08/13/tips-for-parents-children-with-pku-entering-nursery-or-school/

Fidika, A., Salewski, C., Goldbeck, L. (2013). Quality of life among parents of children with phenylketonuria (PKU). *Health and Quality of Life Outcomes, 11*, Article 54.

Morawska, A., Mitchell, A. E., Etel, E., Kirby, G., McGill, J., Roman, D., & Inwood, A. (2019). Psychosocial functioning with phenylketonuria: Relationships between quality of life and parenting indicators. *Child: Care, health and development, 46*(1), 56–65.

Trahms, C. M., & Luce, P. (2003). *New Parents' Guide to PKU.* https://depts.washington.edu/pku/pdfs/New_Parents_Guide_03.pdf

References

Adolph, K. E., Cole, W. G., & Vereijken, B. (2015). Intra-individual variability in the development of motor skills in childhood. In M. Diehl, K. Hooker, & M. Sliwinski (Eds.), *Handbook of intra-individual variability across the lifespan.* Routledge.

Bedford, H., Walton, S., & Ahn, J. (2013). *Measures of child development: A review.* UCL.

Eldred, K., & Darrah, J. (2010). Using cluster analysis to interpret the variability of gross motor scores of children with typical development. *Physical Therapy, 90*(10), 1510–1518. https://doi.org/10.2522/ptj.20090308

Hadders-Algra, M. (2010). Variation and variability: Key words in human motor development. *Physical Therapy, 90*(12), 1823–1837. https://doi.org/10.2522/ptj.20100006

Smith, L. B., & Thelen, E. (1993). *A dynamic systems approach to development.* Bradford Books.

Touwen, B. C. L. (1993). How normal is variable, or how variable is normal? *Early Human Development, 34*(1-2), 1–12. https://doi.org/10.1016/0378-3782(93)90035-S

van Dijk, M., & van Geert, P. (2014). The nature and meaning of intraindividual variability in development in the early life span. In M. Diehl, K. Hooker, & M. Sliwinski (Eds.), *Handbook of intraindividual variability across the life span* (pp. 37–58). Routledge.

Woolf, L. I., Griffiths, R., & Moncrieff, A. (1955). Treatment of phenylketonuria with a diet low in phenylalanine. *British Medical Journal, 1*(57), 31–45. https://doi.org/10.1136/bmj.1.4905.57

Zone 5

Zone 5: Children With Variability in Typical Development	
Chapter 17	Leo: A Child With Variability Above the Range of Typical Development
Chapter 18	James: A Child With Variability Within the Range of Typical Development

Chapter 17

Leo: A Child With Variability Above the Range of Typical Development

Paul O'Callaghan and Inna Polianska

The Context

Leo was attending a large international school of around 1,700 students in Saudi Arabia. The school was situated in a university compound, with both parents employed at the university – in research and in university administration. The family had moved to Saudi Arabia in 2017, to take up employment at the university. Both parents had been born in Brazil, and they spoke both English and Portuguese at home. Leo was the first born of two and demonstrated remarkable abilities from an early age (e.g., he was able to read books containing multisyllabic words by age 3 years and could count up to 1,000 at 4 years).

Leo was referred to the school psychologist during his final year of kindergarten to ascertain if he should be promoted early to Grade 1. The assessment, which was conducted in October and November 2019, when Leo was 5 years 8 months, sought to identify Leo's cognitive ability (Wechsler Pre-School and Primary Scale of Intelligence for Children, 4th edition; Wechsler, 2013), his literacy and numeracy attainments (Wechsler Individual Achievement Test, 3rd edition; Wechsler, 2009), and his social-emotional development (Griffiths Scales of Child Development, 3rd edition) to firstly understand his current level of functioning, and secondly to use this data to advise the school administration on whether grade promotion was warranted, or not.

In particular, the Griffiths III was chosen to provide a standardized measure of behavioral and emotional maturity – as concerns had been expressed in the past from staff about Leo's behavior and whether he had the social and emotional maturity to be successful in a higher grade.

The Child

Leo was born in Brazil in February 2014. When he was born, his mother took a career break, to care for him at home. After his first birthday, Leo was enrolled in a local English speaking playgroup in Rio de Janeiro. In 2017, his parents moved to Saudi Arabia for work, and Leo enrolled in kindergarten 1 (K1) in August 2017, when he was three and a half years old.

In his first year in kindergarten, Leo had presented with behavioral challenges, including running away from staff, physical aggression (kicking, pushing, spitting, and throwing objects), verbal aggression (e.g., shouting at peers and adults), noncompliance with staff directives, and not following toileting expectations during outside play. Since then, both school and home had implemented specific strategies to support his behavioral development. These are indicated in Table 17.1 below.

Table 17.1. Matrix of specific strategies to support behavioral development

Acknowledgement for handling frustration well	Teaching the stop, think, do routine	Offering choice during free play	Visual aids (e.g., cloud puppet)
1:1 Time with a counselor	Reduced screen time at home	Deep breathing sessions	Using a jar of locks and number bonds
Provision of more challenging material	Individual workstation	Library visits	Access to complex puzzles and dominoes
Helping with whole school announcements	Natural consequences	Emails home for positive behavior	Assisting with young student's reading

In kindergarten, Leo was case managed by the gifted and talented coordinator, who provided teacher and parent consultation support. The school counselor also supported him in identifying his feelings and practicing relaxation strategies for when he was upset. At the time of the assessment, Leo's interests included the states of America, countries and capitals of the world, flags of the world, and mathematical series.

Check Your Progress

- How did Leo behave in kindergarten?
- What strategies were put in place to support him?

The Condition

Given the evidence suggesting broadly negative effects of grade retention on motivation (Kretschmann et al., 2019), academics (Abbott et al., 2010), and school completion (Hughes et al., 2018), it is hardly surprising that many schools are cautious about grade promotion for students with exceptional ability. After all, if one policy to separate struggling students from their classmates is broadly considered to be ineffective (Range et al., 2011), surely a policy to separate exceptionally strong students from their classmates is also questionable.

Also, weighing heavily on schools is the fear of "opening the floodgates" to emboldened parents and teachers who would start to advocate for the same approach for other children in the school, while often lacking the context or any basis for an accurate comparison with the exceptionally able child who was promoted. Then there are legitimate concerns about social-emotional effects of placing chronologically younger children with older peers, and their difficulties in integrating in a new grade level (Bernstein et al., 2020). With the stakes so high for both students and schools, it is even more crucial, then, that research evidence becomes the primary driver of decision making.

A recently published 35-year longitudinal study of the psychological effects of academic acceleration of over 1,500 intellectually precocious students (Bernstein et al., 2020) found no covariance between academic acceleration and long-term psychological well-being. In fact, the mental health of both accelerated and nonaccelerated gifted students was similar and higher than that of the normal population. This study is significant in that it measures long-term health outcomes over more than 3 decades, and contrary to some widely held beliefs, offers the most definitive evidence to date that grade promotion does not have a deleterious effect on mental health or psychological well-being.

Another longitudinal study that interviewed 88 adults who were identified as gifted while at school (Perrone et al., 2010) to ascertain their views about advanced classes and gifted programs, reported that 88% would support advanced placements for their children if it were recommended by the school. Of course, not all schools think similarly about this topic, and not all children are likely to be accelerated even if they are gifted. In an analysis and comparison of the National Education Longitudinal Study of 1988 (NELS:88) and the Education Longitudinal Study of 2002 (ELS:2002), Wells and colleagues (2009) found that other things being equal, female students, Asian Americans, and students living in the US east or west coast were more likely to be grade accelerated. However, when grade accelerated students were compared with older classmates of similar achievement who were not accelerated, accelerated students showed greater gains in achievement than nonaccelerated students.

With evidence pointing to overall positive academic benefits, and no overall negative social-emotional impacts to acceleration, it is now up to each school to obtain a global profile of each student being considered for acceleration, to understand better both their academic and their social, emotional, and behavioral profile. Obtaining valid and reliable data on younger students' social, emotional, and behavioral development is a challenge, and so Griffiths III with its standardized score, on Subscale D (personal-social-emotional), was just the assessment needed to provide up-to-date information on Leo's current social and emotional needs.

Check Your Progress

- What is the evidence that grade acceleration may help gifted students?
- How did Victor show progress after the intervention?

The Consultation

Observation

Leo was observed during both a physical education (PE) class and a math lesson in October 2019. During his PE class, he sat at his place on the mat. He was attentive and focused on what his teacher was saying. He followed the teacher's instructions and moved between stations without difficulty. He waited his turn and interacted well with his peers, while waiting to have his turn at the exercise station. He then transitioned without difficulty to his classroom after the PE lesson.

During the math class, he was the only student in the class able to identify a math category (odd numbers). He was the first student to know the number that the teacher was thinking of and able to explain that the number the teacher had chosen was part of the Fibonacci series. While his peers were identifying numbers smaller than 100 and adding numbers smaller than 10, Leo was completing calculations involving numbers greater than 1,000. During class, he responded immediately to classroom tidy-up cues, completing his tasks promptly, transitioned well between tasks, and followed all of the instructions given by his teacher. Although not evident in this current observation, in the past, school staff had identified some perfectionist traits, which staff addressed in an empathetic but consistent manner, allowing choice where possible and being firm in the behavioral expectations that Leo needed to abide by in the school.

Leo came willingly to the assessment room and engaged well throughout the assessment. However, he did become more disengaged over time, and negotiation was required to build in breaks to complete all of the subtests required. It was clear that Leo had particular ability in the visual-spatial tasks (e.g., Block Design) and was disappointed when he had completed all of the items in the subtest, and there were no more left. Once, when redirected to sit properly, he initially did not engage and curled up on the couch. However, after some selective ignoring, and telling Leo we would only start when he was ready, the assessment proceeded without difficulty.

Explanation of Observations With Leo

Observation in class indicated a student who presents with significant math skills, far beyond what his peers were currently learning. Also, pleasing progress was observed in his ability to adhere to classroom expectations and interact appropriately with both peers and school staff. At times during the assessment, Leo exhibited a reticence to complete tasks, particularly tasks he did not find motivating (e.g., a reading test); however, with rest breaks, encouragement, and a clear explanation of the tasks he had to complete, he was able to complete everything required of him.

Cognitive Assessment

Leo's thinking and reasoning (cognitive) skills were assessed using the Wechsler Pre-School and Primary Scale of Intelligence for Children, 4th edition (WPPSI-IV). The WPPSI measures verbal and visual-spatial reasoning skills, ability to solve novel problems (fluid reasoning), ability to hold and manipulate information in memory (working memory), and speed of visual discrimination and task attention (processing speed). A full-scale IQ score was also calculated, which was considered to be the most representative indicator of Leo's current general intellectual functioning. These results are shown in Table 17.2 below.

Table 17.2. Wechsler Pre-School and Primary Scale of Intelligence for Children, 4th edition (WPPSI-IV) results for Leo

Composite scores	Standard score	Confidence interval (95%)	Percentile rank	Descriptor
Verbal comprehension (information, similarities)	140	131–144	99.6	Well above average
Visual spatial skills (block design subtest)	145		99.9	Well above average
Fluid reasoning skills (matrix reasoning subtest)	130		98	Well above average
Working memory subtest (picture memory subtest)	135		99	Well above average
Processing speed subtest (bug search subtest)	120		91	Above average
Full scale IQ score	144	137–148	99.8	Well above average

Explanation of Leo's Cognitive Scores

Leo's overall ability (standard score 137–148) fell within the gifted range. This score is found in about one in 500 students Leo's age and is one of the highest overall ability scores ever recorded in the school psychologist's ten years of practice. As confirmed by classroom observation and teacher reporting, and in line with students of exceptional ability, Leo enjoyed exploring intricate concepts (replicating complex shapes with blocks), was highly curious (he wanted to know why the assessment was taking place and what it measured), and engaged in abstract and complex reasoning (complex matrix problem solving). He demonstrated a rich vocabulary for a 5-year-old (e.g., he could name planets, compass directions, and oceans) and showed learning at a rate significantly faster than his chronological-age peers.

Attainment and Achievement Assessment

Leo's literacy and numeracy skills were assessed using the Wechsler Individual Achievement Test (WIAT-III). This individually administered test assesses academic skills and gives a profile of academic strengths and weaknesses. Standard scores between 85 and 115 are average.

Caveat: due to Leo's young age, there were no literacy norms available for his age, and so literacy norms of students at the beginning of Grade 1 were used instead. Thus, all of Leo's literacy scores were an underestimation of what would be expected given his current chronological age. His numeracy scores, however, were age-appropriate comparisons. These results are shown in Table 17.3 below.

Table 17.3. Wechsler Individual Achievement Test (WIAT-III) results for Leo

Area	Standard score	Confidence interval (95%)	Percentile rank	Descriptor
Literacy assessments				
Reading comprehension*	> 114	> 106–122	> 82	Average
Word reading*	> 129	> 125–133	> 97	Above average
Spelling*	> 111	> 102–120	> 77	Average
Numeracy assessments				
Math problem solving	160	158 Ceiling	99.9	Well above average
Numerical operations	160	158 Ceiling	99.9	Well above average

Note. *Expected to be an underestimation of Leo's age-appropriate literacy scores, since age norms corresponding to Leo's age were not available for the literacy subtests administered.

Explanation of Leo's Achievement and Attainment Scores

Leo scored in the well-above-average range in both mathematical reasoning and arithmetic computation, with scores commonly found in approximately 1 in 1,000 students. He was able to read graphs, read analogue time, identify place numbers, answer probability questions, and solve fraction problems. Meanwhile, all of his literacy scores were above average for Grade 1. He could read three- and four-syllable words (e.g., "playfully" and "ridiculous") and read words with silent letters (e.g., "crumb" and "rhyme"). He could also extract meaning from text (e.g., answering information questions) and deduce meaning from context (e.g., applying information from a text to a particular scenario).

Personal-Social-Emotional Assessment

Leo's self-care, self-regulation, and social and peer interaction skills (personal-social-emotional skills) were assessed using the Griffiths Scales of Child Development, 3rd edition (Griffiths III). Again, some caution must be observed in interpreting Leo's score, due to potential ceiling effects arising from his age being at the uppermost limit of the age range for the Griffiths III assessment. These results are shown in Table 17.4 below.

Table 17.4. Griffiths Scales of Child Development, 3rd edition (Griffiths III): Personal-social-emotional subscale results for Leo

Subscale	Development quotient	Confidence interval (95%)	Percentile	Descriptor
Subscale D	94	93–97	36%	Average

Explanation of Leo's Personal-Social-Emotional Scores

Leo could calm himself if frustrated, had a best friend, and had largely independent eating, toileting, and dressing skills. He was able to identify emotions (including disgust), reason morally, understand the reasons for people's feelings, understand other people's perspectives (theory of mind), and assert himself appropriately in social situations. Leo's score on the personal-social-emotional subscale on Griffiths III was age-appropriate and supported the teacher's reporting of no significant behavioral, emotional, or social concerns in school at that time.

Check Your Progress

- Which tests were used to confirm Leo's cognitive ability?
- Why was Subscale D of the Griffiths III used in conjunction with other tests?

Connecting the Dots

Leo was a 5-year-old student in his final year of kindergarten at a large international school in Saudi Arabia. In September 2019, following parental discussions, a request was made to assess Leo's cognitive, math, and numeracy attainments to better understand his current level of functioning and how best to support his learning at school.

School staff consultation identified both significant high ability traits as well as some behavioral challenges (e.g., aggression, difficulty following school expectations, inappropriate behavior, etc.), which appeared to have lessened over time as Leo had matured.

Observation indicated a student who presented with significant ability, who could follow classroom expectations and interact appropriately with both peers and school staff.

Cognitive assessment on the WPPSI-IV indicated a full-scale IQ score falling in the gifted range (standard score 137–148). Although some caution must be observed in drawing too many conclusions from this first assessment given Leo's age and the greater variability in cognitive scores among young children; nevertheless, it did indicate particularly high ability present in approximately 1 in 100 to 1 in 500 students of Leo's age.

Due to Leo's age, literacy norms were only available for Grade 1, but assessment indicated above average literacy attainments for Grade 1. Meanwhile, his math attainments were in the highest range possible on the test and indicated scores found in approximately 1 in 1,000 students.

Personal-social-emotional skills assessment using Griffiths III Subscale D found at least average personal-social-emotional skills, with strengths noted in his ability to understand other people's perspectives (theory of mind), peer interaction skills, and age-appropriate self-help skills.

Key Strengths and Needs

- Leo benefits from daily practice at progressively more challenging math and reading tasks, with opportunities to work independently on his areas of interest.
- Leo needs opportunities to work and socialize with like-minded peers.
- Leo requires lessons which are differentiated in quantity, pace, review time, and content presentation (Rogers, 2007).
- Finally, Leo needs both grade-level and subject-level acceleration to support his learning at school.

Charting a Plan

The following strategies were designed to support Leo's learning in the future:

- Learning inside the classroom: Leo needs daily practice at progressively more challenging math and reading tasks, with lessons differentiated in quantity, pace, review time (Leo would require less review time to master a concept than many of his peers), and forms of content presentation. Where possible, working with like-minded peers is of help to him.
- Learning outside the classroom: Children with Leo's abilities often seek complexity and show interest in topics and learning outside the classroom. Nurturing these interests through online programs (e.g., Khan Academy, Raz Kids, etc.) and trips to museums and science labs and other places of interest allows Leo to develop his domains of specialist interest.
- Bibliotherapy: Leo displays many of the social and emotional characteristics associated with giftedness. Some books that help him develop his awareness of his developing so-

cial and cognitive skills included *The Gifted Kid Book Series* by Gloria van Donge, *Big Ideas for Curious Minds* by the School of Life, and *The Bird and The Elephant* by Dominic Smith.
- Cultivating Leo's areas of interest: Leo thrives when given opportunities to work independently in his current area of interest. The opportunity to reach or learn more about his area of expertise is a powerful motivator to complete tasks that are less motivating.
- Acceleration: Acting on the evidence of the assessment data, and with parental support, the school provides both grade-level and subject-level acceleration to support Leo's learning at school.
- Counseling support: Leo continues to benefit from opportunities for 1:1 support with his counselor to help him develop self-regulation skills and resolve any peer conflicts that might have arise.

Check Your Progress

- Where will the plan take place?

Conclusion

In early December 2019, the school administration agreed to promote Leo to Grade 1. However, within months of joining Grade 1, the COVID-19 pandemic struck, and much of Leo's Grade 1 year was spent in distance learning. He is now currently in Grade 2 and accesses enrichment math sessions with the school's new talent and enrichment coordinator. He also sees the elementary school counselor for a 6-week block of individual support targeting emotional regulation (e.g., body awareness of different emotions, identifying anger triggers, learning about his emotional thermometer, and practicing calming techniques).

This case study has shown how a Griffiths III assessment can be integrated alongside other cognitive, literacy, and numeracy assessments to provide a rich and comprehensive student profile. This assessment has also challenged our thinking about who we predominantly use the Griffiths III assessment with. Is Griffiths III primarily an assessment for children presenting with global developmental delay, language delays, and motor challenges? What about those with exceptional abilities – a population that can be overlooked in schools – due to their strong academic performance?

The chapter has also demonstrated *asynchronous development*' (Silverman, 1997) and how gifted children's development is often uneven, with areas of great strength (e.g., verbal and nonverbal reasoning) and areas of average ability (processing speed, personal-social-emotional skills). Furthermore, this case has shown the value of including social-emotional measures in all comprehensive assessments, because gifted children can still warrant grade promotion, even if their emotional maturity is not as advanced as their cognitive and academic skills.

Discussion Questions

- How much weight should schools give to personal-social-emotional skills when considering grade promotion?
- What additional strategies would you recommend that home and school put in place to support Leo if he had scored in the below average range on Subscale D?
- What additional assessments of social, emotional, and behavioral development might have been used by the school to validate the finding on Subscale D?
- Subscale D is comprised of diverse skills (e.g., theory of mind vs. self-care skills). Would a low score on the theory of mind questions be a better predictor of potential adjustment challenges than a low score on self-care skills (e.g., eating, dressing, toileting, etc.)?
- What are the pros and cons of using multiple different assessments (e.g., WIPPSI-IV, WIAT-III, Griffiths III) vs. using all the subscales of just one assessment (e.g., Griffiths III)?

References

Abbott, M., Wills, H., Greenwood, C. R., Kamps, D., Heitzman-Powell, L., & Selig, J. (2010). The combined effects of grade retention and targeted small-group intervention on students' literacy outcomes. *Reading & Writing Quarterly, 26*(1), 4–25. https://doi.org/10.1080/10573560903396876

Bernstein, B. O., Lubinski, D., & Benbow, C. P. (2020). Academic acceleration in gifted youth and fruitless concerns regarding psychological well-being: A 35-year longitudinal study. *Journal of Educational Psychology, 113*(4), 830–845.https://doi.org/10.1037/edu0000500

Hughes, J. N., West, S. G., Kim, H., & Bauer, S. S. (2018). Effect of early grade retention on school completion: A prospective study. *Journal of Educational Psychology, 110*(7), 974–991. https://doi.org/10.1037/edu0000243

Kretschmann, J., Vock, M., Lüdtke, O., Jansen, M., & Gronostaj, A. (2019). Effects of grade retention on students' motivation: A longitudinal study over 3 years of secondary school. *Journal of Educational Psychology, 111*(8), 1432–1446. https://doi.org/10.1037/edu0000353

Perrone, K. M., Wright, S. L., Ksiazak, T. M., Crane, A. L., & Vannatter, A. (2010). Looking back on lessons learned: Gifted adults reflect on their experiences in advanced classes. *Roeper Review, 32*(2), 127–139. https://doi.org/10.1080/02783191003587918

Range, B., Dougan, K., & Pijanowski, J. (2011). Rethinking grade retention and academic redshirting: Helping school administrators make sense of what works. *International Journal of Educational Leadership Preparation, 6*(2), n2.

Rogers, K. B. (2007). Lessons learned about educating the gifted and talented: A synthesis of the research on educational practice. *Gifted Child Quarterly, 51*(4), 382–396. https://doi.org/10.1177/0016986207306324

Silverman, L. K. (1997). The construct of asynchronous development. *Peabody Journal of Education, 72*(3-4), 36–58. https://doi.org/10.1207/s15327930pje7203&4_3

Wechsler, D. (2009). *Wechsler Individual Achievement Test (WIAT-III)* (3rd ed.). Pearson, Psychological Corporation.

Wechsler, D. (2013). *Wechsler Pre-school and primary scale of intelligence for children (WPPSI-IV)* (4th ed.). Pearson, Psychological Corporation.

Wells, R., Lohman, D., & Marron, M. (2009). What factors are associated with grade acceleration? An analysis and comparison of two U.S. databases. *Journal of Advanced Academics, 20*(2), 248–273. https://doi.org/10.1177/1932202X0902000203

Chapter 18

James: A Child With Variability Within the Range of Typical Development

Paula McAlinden

The Context

I worked as a consultant community pediatrician and clinical director for many years in the Southern Health & Social Care Trust in Northern Ireland. The main clinical components of my post were in developmental assessments, where I used the Griffiths Scales routinely. I worked closely with a range of other health care professionals, schools, and educational psychologists, with our primary aim being to help each child achieve their optimum potential, though close collaboration and with the best interests of the child as our primary goal.

In this role, I had the opportunity to work with children and their families from when they initially presented and then as they moved first through primary, then postprimary schools. This allowed me to form extended clinical relationships with the children and their families, and as part of this process and ongoing review, to gain an insight into how the various difficulties the children encountered affected not only themselves but also their parents and siblings.

The case study described here is that of a child who presented with fatigue and poor attention linked to a congenital cardiac condition. While his overall clinical development was normal, closer analysis identified a *specific learning difficulty* (SLD), which had caused both him and his family increasing challenges as he progressed within his schooling, with significant effects on his self-esteem and emotional well-being.

More specifically, this case study is presented to illustrate how Griffiths III can be used to help with the early identification of an SLD in a little boy who while having some medical issues was essentially otherwise showing normal development. The results of his Griffiths III assessment and the ongoing efforts by his mother to ensure his SLD was recognized helped contribute to James' achievements in school, and also reduced the potential social-emotional difficulties he might have experienced due to low mood and self-esteem, as he was very aware of his difficulties with graphomotor tasks. The case study charts the Griffiths III assessment with subsequent plans and linked actions.

The Child

James was born by elective cesarean section at 39 weeks of gestation; he developed *transient tachypnea of newborns* in the neonatal period and required observation in the Special

Care Baby Unit for 36 hrs from day 2 to 4. His birth weight was 3,800 g (8 lb 6 oz), and his Apgar scores were 8 at 1 minute and 9 at 5 minutes. James had been noted to have a cardiac murmur in his neonatal period, but this seemed to have settled by age 12 weeks, so no specification investigations were carried out at that stage. He was noted again to have a cardiac murmur at GP review when aged 18 months. James was then referred to a pediatric cardiologist for further investigation, who subsequently diagnosed him as having a *coarctation of his aorta* when aged 2 years. He experienced increasing problems with fatigue in the spring and summer when he was 3 years old and required a balloon angioplasty of his coarctation. Following his cardiac catheterization, James' parents were advised he did not need to be restricted in any physical activity. James was to continue to require regular cardiology reviews into adulthood.

James was seen for assessment aged 4 years 6 months (Year 2 of his formal schooling), as he was experiencing significant fatigue with exercise and tired early within the school day. This was variable, but even after a good night's sleep he could be tired in school by 10:00 a.m. James was also noted at the time to have poor attention and concentration and some fine motor difficulties which affected his writing; these difficulties are often associated with coarctation of the aorta. In school, James required help to keep him focused on activities and frequent breaks while working.

The Condition

James' mother had had no specific concerns about his development preschool. He did not crawl until almost 8 months but walked at 14 months. He had a vocabulary of 20+ words at his 18-month health visitor assessment. While he greatly enjoyed building activities, he was less keen on coloring in and painting. James had both coarctation of the aorta and a *bicuspid aortic valve*. Coarctation of the Aorta is a narrowing of the artery that carries blood from the heart to the head and body. James had had his narrowing stretched at 3 years old using a nonsurgical technique cardiac catheterization. A bicuspid aortic valve means that the aortic valve has only two flaps instead of the normal three.

Various studies have shown that both cyanotic and acyanotic conditions including coarctation of the aorta are associated with specific sensorimotor delays, regardless of the method of correction (McCusker et al., 2007). Studies have shown that overall, such children have intelligence scores that fall within the normal range (Spijkerboer et al., 2008). Prior to the early 1980s, it was uncommon for children with complex congenital heart disease (CHD) to survive into later childhood, but subsequent developments in congenital cardiac surgery, interventional cardiac catheterization, echocardiography, and intensive care medicine have combined to improve survival rates of these children. Approximately half of those children with complex CHD who survive have complex neurodevelopmental disorders, which include mild cognitive impairment, expressive speech and language abnormalities, learning disabilities, impaired visual-spatial and visual-motor skills, and attention-deficit/hyperactivity disorders (ADHD; Wernovsky & Licht, 2016). The child featured in this case study had an SLD – namely, *dysgraphia*. Generally, dysgraphia refers to extremely poor handwriting, and while it can occur in isolation, it can also be associated with dyslexia and in this case a congenital cardiac problem.

Check Your Progress

- What types of developmental difficulty are associated with congenital heart disease?

The Consultation

Griffiths III was initially used to assess James' development when he was aged 4 years 6 months. The assessment was undertaken in a single session, but it was immediately clear that James was extremely active and restless and that he struggled to sit back on his chair and to follow the examiner's instructions. However, once he was involved with a particular activity, he was able to focus and concentrate appropriately on that activity.

Subscale A

James correctly completed both object hunt items and also all of the memory house items including the incidental memory task. He greatly enjoyed timed activities completing the six-hole formboard in 11 seconds, the eleven-hole formboard in 33 seconds, and the patternmaking in 31 seconds. James was also able to repeat four but not five-digit numbers or a sequence of numbers reversed. He built a bridge and a castle and also completed the train puzzle. He identified five of the six spot-the-difference items. He drew a Stage 2 person and was able to do the first of two picture arrangement items. James very much enjoyed these activities, and he performed many tasks at the level of a child up to 12 months older than he was.

Subscale B

James named 16 objects and correctly defined the use of 10 of these. He named all 8 of the activity picture cards and understood complex sentences. He repeated a 10- but not a 16-word sentence, and was able to follow positional words and two-step instructions. While not yet able to tell a story about the large picture, James used three descriptive sentences to describe the picture. He understood all three of the opposites, similarities, and difference items. He took part in a short conversation about his interest in computers and also correctly defined two-word definition items. James scored at an age-appropriate level in his language performance, and this may have been influenced by his ability to listen fully to longer instructions.

Subscale C

James was left-handed and had an immature pencil grip. He drew a Stage 1 circle and cross and a Stage 2 person and could also write his first name. He put 12 pegs into the peg board in 49 seconds. He was able to bolt two construction pieces together, and his mother reported he loved Lego- and Meccano-type activities. He was not able to complete any of the trail making tasks or the dot-to-dot activities, but he was able to do up three buttons and fold a square of paper twice. James correctly imitated a sequential finger item. While James appeared to achieve an age-appropriate level of result for his eye and hand coordination overall, closer analysis showed he had particular difficulties with his graphomotor skills, which were below those expected of a child of his age.

Subscale D

James tended to be a sociable boy and had a best friend in school. He identified five of six facial expressions and also understood reasons for people's feelings. He understood the rules of games. He correctly completed the perspective-taking cards and also the false belief test but not the beach perspective-taking task. He responded correctly to two of the moral reasoning questions and for one of the socially assertive questions. James' mother reported that he was able to dress himself except for difficult fastenings and was fully toilet trained. He was also able to eat a meal neatly. James' scores on the personal-social-emotional subscale confirmed that his social skills and his self-care skills were age appropriate.

Subscale E

James enjoyed moving around for the gross motor tasks. He could stand on one leg for 6 seconds and do a three-star jump sequence but could not yet do a hop, jump sequence. James was able to walk along a tape for over 1 m and precisely heel-to-toe forward along a 1.5-m (approximately five-foot) tape. He could however not walk backwards. He was able to run fast and kicked the short tennis ball through a "goal" of bricks. He was also able to bounce and catch the short tennis ball. James performed above his developmental age on the gross motor subscale. Table 18.1 below indicates James' scores on all five subscales of Griffiths III.

Table 18.1. James' scores on Griffiths III

Subscale	Raw score	Developmental age (months)	Scaled score	Development quotient (DQ)	Confidence interval (95%)	Percentile	Stanine
Subscale A	59	67	15	126	123–129	95	8
Subscale B	57	56	11	104	103–105	59	6
Subscale C	57	55	11	103	102–104	56	5
Subscale D	60	60	12	110	109–112	73	6
Subscale E	57	62	13	113	110–115	78	7
General development	58	60	13	114	113–116	81	7

Using the base rates obtained during the standardization of Griffiths III, the maximum difference of 4 in the subscale scaled scores confirmed that there was no significant difference between subscale scores. The use of a development quotient (DQ) was also appropriate.

Check Your Progress

- What did the assessment show?

Connecting the Dots

James was born with complex congenital heart disease which was partially corrected at 3 years old. He was assessed at age 4 years because of concerns about significant fatigue with exercise and tiredness early within the school day. James was noted at the time to have poor attention and concentration and poor focus on activities, together with some fine motor difficulties which affected his writing.

Overall, James scored very highly on his Griffiths III assessment particularly on the foundations of learning, personal-emotional-social, and gross motor subscales. All of his scores were above or equal to those for his developmental age and DQ including those for Language and eye and hand coordination. However, a closer analysis of the constructs within the eye and hand coordination subscale confirmed that while James did very well with construction-type tasks, his graphomotor skills were delayed, his writing was immature, he struggled to draw more than basic shapes or to complete dot-to-dot and trail activities, and in this area his skills were significantly below those expected for a child of his age.

The occupational therapist noted that while easily distracted, James attended well in a one-to-one situation, but with frequent breaks over a 3-hr period. She concluded that he was a child with considerable ability who had some difficulty with handwriting and attention in class, probably due to a mild sensorimotor delay.

When James was 7 years 8 months, his parents arranged a private psychology assessment. The psychologist saw James on two consecutive days to aid his concentration and to minimize the effects of fatigue. While James was willing to participate throughout both sessions, his cooperation waned slightly as his energy decreased. He needed to position himself comfortably with his body against a prop before he could focus his attention, and he also needed to move frequently. His responses to vocabulary items, social comprehension item, and items which required contrasting and comparing objects and even abstract concepts, showed an advance level of analytical cognitive skill for his age. Overall, James' mathematical thinking and problem-solving skills appeared to be at a good average level for his age, but he preferred to solve mathematical problem orally. His writing was below the standard expected for his age, and he reversed his writing of the letters "j," "p," and "q," and hesitated over "b" and "d." His writing was often above the line rather than on it, and he confused homonyms ("write" and "right"). It was obvious that his motivation for written tasks was poor.

The results of psychometric evaluation indicated that James had an SLD in written literacy skills, with features of dysgraphia, as a child with above-average intellectual ability. His oral and aural skills were well above average for his age. He demonstrated variable concentration both due to his variable energy levels and partly due to his poor motivation for written tasks.

An assessment by an occupational therapist was recommended, and it was also suggested that James would benefit from additional support within the school classroom to keep him focused on activities and to maximize his learning at the times of the school day when his energy was best. It was also suggested that James would benefit from assistance to help his reading and stimulation of his fine motor skills including his writing. James was a popular boy who did not have behavioral difficulties.

Check Your Progress

- What are the reasons for James' difficulties?

Charting a Plan

No specific intervention was available at that time to address his difficulties with fatigability. The psychologist made a number of focused recommendations involving close liaison with his school:

- Trying to reduce the quantity of written tasks that James was asked to do.
- Giving James plenty of time to take down his homework perhaps by displaying it on a white board in the morning or sending this home electronically.
- Providing James with help with his spelling.
- Teaching James to touch type as his hands got stronger – this helped with spelling and also the legibility and speed of written work. In the interim he continued working to improve his handwriting.
- Giving James breaks between academic tasks and also movement breaks.
- Trying to keep his learning environment as visually and auditorily neutral and distraction-free as possible.

The occupational therapist recommended that he should sit close to the teacher in a quiet area of his classroom, and she also provided both a handwriting and a sensory-seeking program for use in school.

James' parents used a variety of strategies to help with his fine motor difficulties, including carrying out a sensory program at home before he went to school. On weekends, they tried to ensure that they did a lot of family outdoor activities. James went to the breakfast club in his school several days a week, and this gave him time to do a range of activities before settling to the more academic tasks in his school day. He also seemed to benefit from a healthy carbohydrate snack midmorning in school.

Conclusion

Over time James became increasingly aware of his writing difficulties particularly as he progressed in school, and this had a significant effect on his confidence and self-esteem. As the variety of his school subjects increased, he found recording the long essay type answers required by some subjects and languages challenging. His performance was influenced by how individual teachers motivated him and his interest in the subject, overall doing better in mathematics and science subjects. He became a very confident reader and was reading the Harry Potter books and other similar books before his peer group. While he was very motivated by IT activities, he resisted learning to type competently using either traditional or cartoon typing programs.

This case study highlights how an SLD can have a major impact on a child's academic and social performance and the need for such difficulties to be addressed at an early stage in their school career. This is particularly important with the increasing awareness of adolescents to mental health difficulties often associated with low mood and poor self-esteem. It is possible that an earlier assessment by his school's educational psychologist may have ensured earlier additional support within the school setting for James' SLD and helped to reduce his low mood and poor self-esteem.

His mother coincidentally was also a community pediatrician and was aware of how his difficulties impacted on his schoolwork and also his self-esteem and willingness to engage with written activities. James' father conversely struggled to understand the impact of James' congenital heart condition and dysgraphia and was frustrated by what he perceived to be rather his stubborn determination not to engage with his homework. It was a constant challenge to get James to do homework tasks, with homework regularly taking over 2 hrs to complete. He did not respond well to sanctions for work not completed and always needed incentives for written tasks. James had an older sister who was a high academic achiever, and at times she felt upset that James was getting additional attention from their mother.

James' school principal was understanding of his difficulties and tried unsuccessfully to formally obtain additional support for him through the Special Education Code of Practice for him. The ongoing efforts by his mother to ensure his SLD was recognized helped contribute to James' positive achievements in school, and also reduced the potential social-emotional difficulties he might have experienced from low mood and self-esteem, as he was very sensitive of his difficulties with graphomotor tasks.

This case study highlights the importance of looking at the various constructs within each subscale in the Griffiths III assessment for children with relatively typical overall development, to identify specific areas of difficulty so that with appropriate early intervention, the child can achieve their best outcomes. This case study also illustrates how a child with an SLD such as dysgraphia can go unidentified, be academically disadvantaged, and experience more difficulties with their social and emotional well-being.

Discussion Questions

- How will James respond to the increasing challenges of more independent working and increased length of written task as he progresses through school?
- What will the effect be on James of annual changes in his class teacher in primary school?
- What is likely to be the best option for James for his postprimary schooling – comprehensive or grammar school?
- How will James cope with the increased demands of additional subjects in his postprimary schooling – introduction of foreign languages and more essay-type and project work?
- What additional supports including the use of technology might help within the school setting, for both exams and submission of written tasks?
- To what extent might James' dysgraphia affect the choices of his GCSE subjects to help maintain his motivation and results in these exams?
- Is James likely to do best following traditional A level studies post his GCSEs or might alternative educational opportunities such as a BTEC course or an apprenticeship suit his learning style better?
- What are the potential effects of his ongoing writing and attentional difficulties on James' mental health and self-esteem?

References

McCusker, C. G., Doherty, N. N., Molloy, B., Casey, F., Rooney, N., Mulholland, C., Sands, A., Craig, B., & Stewart, M. (2007). Determinants of neurophysical and behavioural outcomes in early childhood survivors of congenital heart disease. *Archives of Disease in Childhood, 92,* e2–e2. https://doi.org/10.1136/adc.2005.092320

Spijkerboer, A. W., Utens, E. M. W. J., Bogers, A. J. J. C., Verhulst, F. C., & Helbing, W. A. (2008). Long-term intellectual functioning and school-related outcomes in children and adolescents after invasive treatment for congenital heart disease. *British Journal of Developmental Psychology, 26*(4), 457–470. https://doi.org/10.1348/026151007X253323

Wernovsky, G., & Licht, D. J. (2016). *Pediatric Critical Care Medicine, 17*(8 Suppl 1), S232–S242. https://doi.org/10.1097/PCC.0000000000000800

Section IV

Best Practice Strategies and Griffiths III

If you take the time to connect the dots,
You can plot the true shape of their genius —
Shining in their darkest hour.

– Donovan Livingston

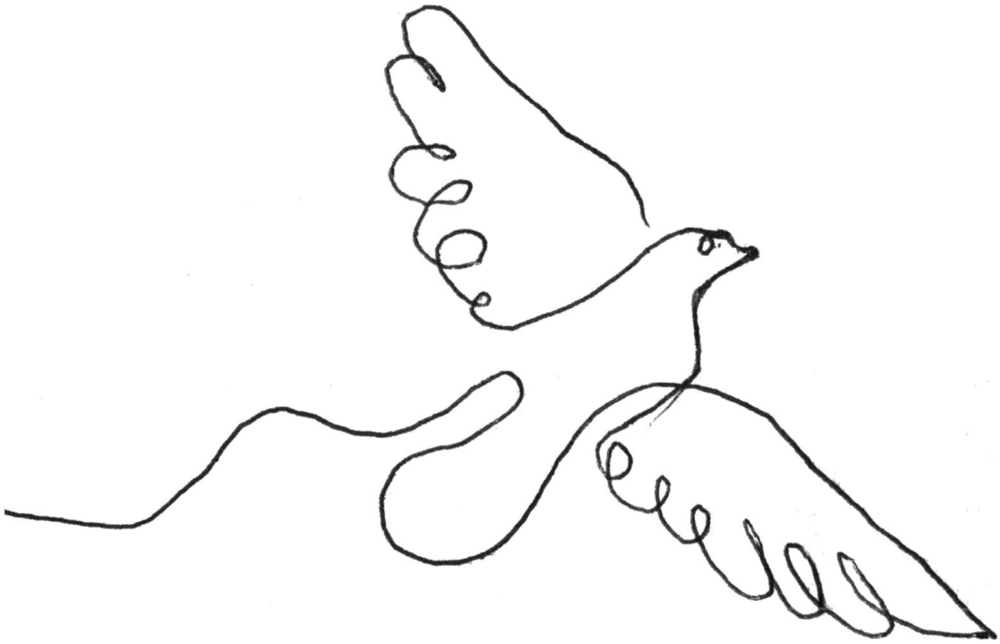

Chapter 19

Griffiths III Best Practice Strategies Emerging From the Cases Presented

Elizabeth Green and Louise Stroud

Perhaps it is time we accept that
psychological sizing up of a human individual
in live function is not as scientifically precise
as sizing up the physical world.

– Phyllis Preston

All of the children depicted in the case studies have their own particular skills and needs. But to see all the colors, there is a need to look beyond the obvious such as to numbers, failures, successes, and functional levels in an assessment.

The tester gains a reflected image of the child, but of what is the image? Blanton and Jaccard (2006) make the pertinent observation that "a researcher who appreciates the gap between a psychological metric and a psychological reality knows to look past a person's score and search for something meaningful" (p. 39). Or to look into the shadows of the mirror: Different images of a child may be held by their parents, carers, teachers, and school, but above all by the child involved. One of the roles of the tester is to use all of the different images of the child to create a meaningful reflection.

All children, including those for whom an assessment is suggested, have needs. Maslow (1943) in his theory of motivation, described the hierarchy of different levels of need (see depiction as a pyramid in Figure 19.1). Self-esteem requires a feeling of accomplishment, so it is important to analyze the barriers to a child's development and look for strategies that may assist the child in all parts of their life – that is, to act as an advocate for the child so that they may reach self-actualization or self-fulfillment.

So, what are the best strategies for searching for something meaningful for a particular child while conducting a developmental assessment? Guidelines exist, some more specific than others and from a range of theoretical viewpoints (American Psychological Association, 2011; Bagnato, 2007; Greenwood &McConnell, 2011; Grisham-Brown et al., 2006; Lebeer et al., 2013; National Research Council, 2008; British Psychological Society, 2015). We have assembled a checklist for practitioners from both the guidelines and the strategies shown in the case studies in this book; this is shown in Box 19.1 below.

"One of my clearest childhood memories is slithering through the tall grass like a snake with my brother and sister" (Nell & Drew, 2013). When you think back on your childhood, what happy play memories come to mind? Adults today tend to think back on their childhood play memories with nostalgia and often call them the "good old days." Memories of joyful and meaningful play experiences help bind families together emotionally, even long after children are grown. Play always has an emotional response attached to it. Without

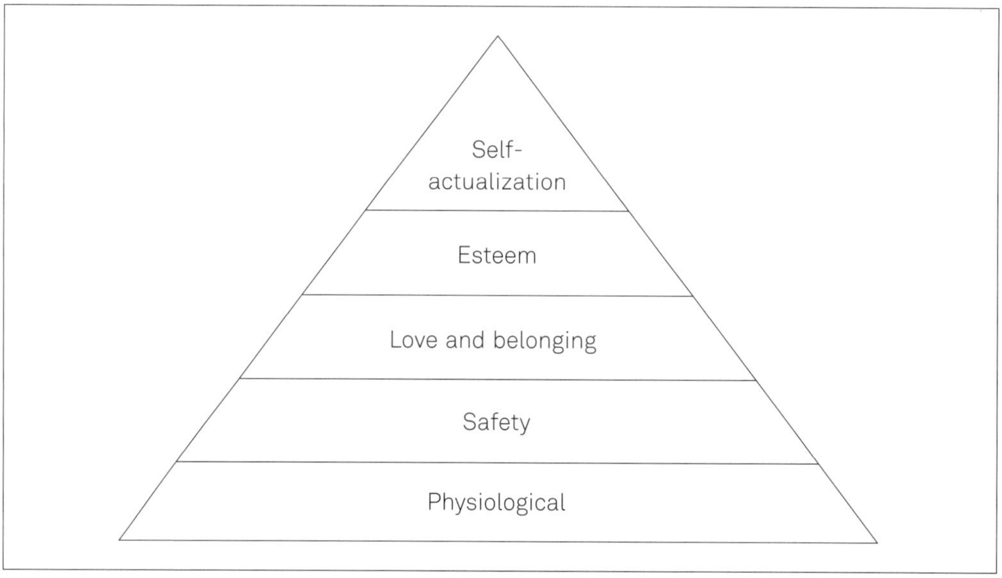

Figure 19.1. A pyramid depiction of Maslow's theory of human need (Maslow, 1943)

this emotional connection, the experience is simply an activity. Enjoyment is the direct result of engaging in play, providing children with a rich experience. And is not that what we want for our children, to develop play memories that will become their own "good old days"?

Box 19.1. Checklist for practitioners reporting standardized developmental tests (Green et al., 2022).

- Depending on the context and goals of assessment and testing, practitioners should use the assessment approach that is most psychometrically sound, fair, comprehensive, and appropriate for children with disabilities.
- Assessment activity should be conducted within a coherent system of medical, educational, and family support services that promote optimal development for all children.
- Define common goals and reframe referral question if necessary.
- Adopt both an interprofessional and family perspective.
- Identify the key environments linked to the child.
- Identify key people for the child and create a positive collaborative relationship.
- Use more than one method of assessment and triangulate the findings and opinions of key people for confirmation of findings.
- Translate standardized measurements and use them in relation to a qualitative description of the child.
- Describe both the strengths and the needs of the child.
- Communicate in plain language and give practical recommendations in relation to the child's individual strengths and needs.
- Consider the barriers to learning for that child and suggest practical options for management.
- Communicate the findings in an inclusive and optimistic way.

Despite the limited snapshot of issues and the literature that has been covered in this case study book, one can be encouraged by the progress that has been made in terms of psychological test development, adaptation, and use around the world in challenging circumstances. It is necessary to celebrate the successes, learn from them (as well as the mistakes made), continue to make progress, and to break new ground in test use, development and cross-cultural adaptation given the world's rich diversity.

References

American Psychological Association. (2011). *Guidelines for assessment and intervention with people with disabilities.* https://www.apa.org/pi/disability/resources/assessment-disabilities.aspx

Bagnato, S. J. (2007). *Authentic assessment for early childhood intervention: Best practices.* Guilford Press.

Blanton, H., & Jaccard, J. I. (2006). Arbitrary metrics in psychology. *American Psychologist, 61,* 27–41. https://doi.org/10.1037/0003-066X.61.1.27

British Psychological Society. (2015). *Guidance on testing with individuals who have intellectual disabilities.*

Green, E. M., Lane, H. M., Cronje, J. H., & Stroud, L. A. (2022). What are the options for reporting development below the floor of a standardized test? Themes from the past 15 years literature. *Global Journal Intellectual and Developmental Disability, 9*(4), 1–9. https://doi.org/10.19080/GJIDD.2022.09.555766

Greenwood, C. R., & McConnell, S. R. (2011). JEI guidelines for manuscripts describing the development and testing of an assessment instrument or measure. *Journal of Early Intervention, 33,* 171–185. https://doi.org/10.1177/1053815111427566

Grisham-Brown, J., Hallam, J., & Brookshire, R. (2006). Using authentic assessment to evidence children's progress toward early learning standards. *Early Childhood Education Journal, 34,* 45–51. https://doi.org/10.1007/s10643-006-0106-y

Lebeer, J., Partanen, P., & Candeias, A. (2013). The need for a more dynamic and ecological assessment of children experiencing barriers to learning to move towards inclusive education: A summary of results of the Daffodil Project. *Erdélyi Pszichológiai Szemle* (Transylvanian Journal of Psychology), *14,* 175–205. https://www.researchgate.net/publication/271838045

Maslow, A. H. (1943). A theory of human motivation. *Psychological Review, 50*(4), 370–396. https://doi.org/10.1037/h0054346

National Research Council. (2008). *Early childhood assessment: Why, what, and how.* National Academies Press.

Nell, M. L., & Drew, W. F. (2013). *From play to practice: Connecting teachers' play to childrens' learning.* The National Association for the Education of Young Children. https://www.naeyc.org/our-work/families/five-essentials-meaningful-play

Chapter 20

A Final Word

Elizabeth Green

The word that comes to mind at the end of this book is *diversity*.

- Diversity of children for whom the use of Griffiths III sheds some light and a route to possible assistance.
- Diversity of parents and socioeconomic backgrounds.
- Diversity of cultures where the children live.
- Diversity of uses of Griffiths III – as a quantitative tool, a qualitative tool, in combination with other assessment tools, one subscale or many subscales, longitudinal assessment.
- Diversity of practitioners performing the assessment.

This has been demonstrated by 14 case studies, which are just a small proportion of case studies carried out in many countries of the world. They are likely to have missed some other aspects, such as the use of a translated *script* to provide uniformity of verbal instruction to the child in their own local language. This works well when the practitioner can read the English of the instructions in the manuals. My confidence in Griffiths III users across the world makes me certain that these case studies show just a fraction of what is possible with such a flexible assessment instrument.

Appendix

Table A1. Case study practice-friendly key concepts grid

Chapter	Advocacy	ADHD	Antenatal diagnosis	ASD	Base rate analysis, subscale significant difference	Choice of educational provision, school entry	Individual education program	Item accommodation (non-standard administration)	Longitudinal assessment	Low socioeconomic status	Multilingual and cultural diversity	Qualitative analysis and quartile charts	School readiness
4	√				√	√	√						√
5	√					√	√	√				√	√
6	√				√	√	√			√	√	√	√
7	√			√	√	√	√			√	√	√	√
8	√			√	√	√	√					√	√
9	√			√	√	√	√			√	√	√	√
10	√			√		√	√		√			√	
11	√	√		√		√	√					√	√
12	√			√					√			√	
13	√					√	√					√	√
14	√	√	√									√	
15	√				√						√		
16	√				√	√	√		√				√
17	√					√					√		
18	√				√		√		√				

Note. ADHD = attention-deficit/ hyperactivity disorder; ASD = autistic spectrum disorder.

Table A2. Use of other additional measures included in case studies

Chapter	ADOS-2	Ages and Stages Questionnaire (ASQ)	Denver II	GMDS-ER	ICF-CY qualifiers	Protocol observation communicative behavior	WIAT-III	WPPSI-IV
4								
5								
6								
7			√			√		
8	√							
9								
10				√	√			
11	√							
12		√						
13								
14								
15								
16								
17							√	√
18								

Note. ADOS-2 = Autism Diagnostic Observation Schedule; GMDS-ER = the Griffiths Mental Development Scales; ICF-CY = *International Classification of Functioning, Disability and Health of Children and Youth* (WHO, 2007); WIAT-III = Wechsler Individual Achievement Test, 3rd edition; WPPSI-IV = Wechsler Pre-School and Primary Scale of Intelligence, 4th edition.

Peer Commentaries

An elegant and concise book which will be very useful for all practitioners of the Griffiths III – both new and experienced users. This excellent compilation of case studies will be a handy resource for the use of Griffiths III with children with different developmental profiles and for assisting in the interpretation of the results.

Soundara Somasundaram, MRCPCH, Associate Specialist in Community Paediatrics, NHS Lothian, Edinburgh, UK

An ounce of experience is worth a ton of theory: The structured psychometric constructs and scales of the Griffiths' profiles have been key to the multidisciplinary practice of developmental pediatrics and neurosciences for decades. The updated version III that helps us assess and support children with a wide range of challenges as well as their families is as important as ever. Context of use is everything and as such, this well-structured casebook on its administration and use in a wide variety of behavioral, physical, and sensory scenarios is extremely helpful and easily accessible to busy clinicians of all professions.

Charles Fairhurst, FRCPCH, Head of Paediatric Neurosciences at Evelina London Children's Hospital, National Clinical Advisor in Paediatric Neurosciences to NHS, London, UK

This is a very welcome publication in the assessment of young children who are confronted daily with developmental milestones. It is the kind of practical book that one mentions to colleagues at every opportunity! Stroud, Green, and their colleagues have carefully selected cases of children which underline why the child-friendly Griffiths III has enjoyed seven decades of use and is the gold standard of providing holistic developmental profiles of both infants and preschool children. This casebook shows the practitioner step-by-step how to conceptualize each unique child and to offer feasible treatment recommendations to help shift the trajectory of a child in real time. As a practitioner and teacher, I was impressed by how reflective the cases are of the actual complex realities that clinicians of young children across the world are faced with. This work stands out due to its sensitive appreciation of the young child and their family, who will directly benefit from their clinician absorbing the wisdom contained in these memorable cases of children with neurodevelopmental needs.

Christine Laidlaw, PhD, Department of Psychology, University of South Africa, Pretoria, South Africa

I am immensely impressed with this book. The case study examples are diverse and discussed in breadth and depth, making this a particularly relevant read for practitioners. The explanation and overview of the Griffiths III, as a child developmental assessment tool, is thorough without being overcomplicating. The Check Your Progress boxes, Discussion Questions, and Key Concepts in the relevant sections keep the reader fully engaged and the quotes and illustrations add beautifully to the overall feel of the book. This is a must read for both novice and seasoned practitioners alike, particularly those with a special interest in the areas of child development and developmental assessments.

Lisa Currin, MA, Department of Psychology, Nelson Mandela University, Port Elizabeth, South Africa